theclinics.com

HEART FAILURE CLINICS

Natriuretic Peptides

GUEST EDITORS
Roger M. Mills, MD
W. H. Wilson Tang, MD
John C. Burnett, Jr, MD

CONSULTING EDITORS
Jagat Narula, MD, PhD
James B. Young, MD

July 2006 • Volume 2 • Number 3

SAUNDERS

An Imprint of Elsevier, Inc.
PHILADELPHIA   LONDON   TORONTO   MONTREAL   SYDNEY   TOKYO

W.B. SAUNDERS COMPANY
A Division of Elsevier Inc.

1600 John F. Kennedy Boulevard. • Suite 1800 • Philadelphia, Pennsylvania 19103-2899

http://www.theclinics.com

HEART FAILURE CLINICS
July 2006
Editor: Karen Sorensen

Volume 2, Number 3
ISSN 1551-7136
ISBN 1-4160-3864-7
978-1-4160-3864-1

Copyright © 2006 Elsevier Inc. All rights reserved. No part of this publication may be reproduced or transmitted in any form or by any means, electronic or mechanical, including photocopy, recording, or any information retrieval system, without written permission from the Publisher.

Single photocopies of single articles may be made for personal use as allowed by national copyright laws. Permission of the publisher and payment of a fee is required for all other photocopying, including multiple or systematic copying, copying for advertising or promotional purposes, resale, and all forms of document delivery. Special rates are available for educational institutions that wish to make photocopies for non-profit educational classroom use. Permissions may be sought directly from Elsevier's Rights Department in Philadelphia, PA, USA at Tel.: (+1) 215-239-3804; Fax: (+1) 215-239-3805; E-mail: healthpermissions@elsevier.com. Requests may also be completed on-line via the Elsevier homepage (http://www.elsevier.com/locate/permissions). In the USA, users may clear permissions and make payments through the Copyright Clearance Center, Inc., 222 Rosewood Drive, Danvers, MA 01923, USA; Tel.: (+1) 978-750-8400; Fax: (+1) 978-750-4744, and in the UK through the Copyright Licensing Agency Rapid Clearance Service (CLARCS), 90, Tottenham Court Road, London W1P 0LP, UK; Tel.: (+44) 171-436-5931; Fax: (+44) 171-436-3986. Other countries may have a local reprographic rights agency for payments.

Reprints: For copies of 100 or more, or articles in this publication, please contact the Commercial Reprints Department, Elsevier Inc., 360 Park Avenue South, New York, New York 10010-1710. Tel.: (+1) 212-633-3813; Fax: (+1) 212-462-1935; e-mail: reprints@elsevier.com.

The ideas and opinions expressed in *Heart Failure Clinics* do not necessarily reflect those of the Publisher. The Publisher does not assume any responsibility for any injury and/or damage to persons or property arising out of or related to any use of the material contained in this periodical. The reader is advised to check the appropriate medical literature and the product information currently provided by the manufacturer of each drug to be administered to verify the dosage, the method and duration of administration, or contraindications. It is the responsibility of the treating physician or other health care professional, relying on independent experience and knowledge of the patient, to determine drug dosages and the best treatment for the patient. Mention of any product in this issue should not be construed as endorsement by the contributors, editors, or the Publisher of the product or manufacturers' claims.

Heart Failure Clinics (ISSN 1551-7136) is published quarterly by Elsevier Inc., 360 Park Avenue South, New York, NY 10010-1710. Months of publication are January, April, July, and October. Business and editorial offices: 1600 John F. Kennedy Boulevard, Suite 1800, Phliadelphia, PA 19103-2899. Customer service office: 6277 Sea Harbor Drive, Orlando, FL 32887-4800. Periodicals postage paid at New York, NY and additional mailing offices. Subscription prices are USD 157 per year for US individuals, USD 260 per year for US institutions, USD 54 per year for US students and residents, USD 189 per year for Canadian individuals, USD 292 per year for Canadian institutions, USD 189 per year for international individuals, USD 292 per year for international institutions and USD 65 per year for foreign students/residents. To receive student and resident rate, orders must be accompanied by name of affiliated institution, date of term, and the *signature* of program/residency coordinator on institution letterhead. Orders will be billed at individual rate until proof of status is received. Foreign air speed delivery is included in all *Clinics* subscription prices. All prices are subject to change without notice. POSTMASTER: Send address changes to *Heart Failure Clinics*, Elsevier Periodicals Customer Service, 6277 Sea Harbor Drive, Orlando, FL 32887-4800. **Customer Service: 1-800-654-2452 (US). From outside of the US, call (+1) 407-345-4000.**

Printed in the United States of America.

Cover artwork courtesy of Umberto M. Jezek.

CONSULTING EDITORS

JAGAT NARULA, MD, PhD, Professor, Medicine; Chief, Division of Cardiology; and Associate Dean, University of California Irvine School of Medicine, Irvine, California

JAMES B. YOUNG, MD, Chairman and Professor, Department of Medicine, Lerner College of Medicine; and George and Linda Kaufman Chair, Cleveland Clinic Foundation, Case Western Reserve University, Cleveland, Ohio

GUEST EDITORS

ROGER M. MILLS, MD, Vice President for Medical Affairs, Scios, Inc., Fremont, California

W.H. WILSON TANG, MD, FACC, Assistant Professor of Medicine, Cleveland Clinic Lerner College of Medicine, Case Western Reserve University; Staff Cardiologist, Section of Heart Failure and Cardiac Transplantation Medicine, Department of Cardiovascular Medicine, Cleveland Clinic, Cleveland, Ohio

JOHN C. BURNETT, JR, MD, Cardiorenal Research Laboratory, Division of Cardiovascular Diseases, Mayo Clinic, Rochester, Minnesota

CONTRIBUTORS

JOHN C. BURNETT, Jr, MD, Professor, Departments of Internal Medicine and Physiology; and Cardiorenal Research Laboratory, Division of Cardiovascular Diseases, Mayo Clinic College of Medicine, Rochester, Minnesota

ALESSANDRO CATALIOTTI, MD, PhD, Assistant Professor of Medicine, Cardiorenal Research Laboratory, Division of Cardiovascular Diseases, Mayo Clinic, Rochester, Minnesota

HORNG H. CHEN, MBBCh, Associate Professor of Medicine, Department of Internal Medicine; and Cardiorenal Research Laboratory, Division of Cardiovascular Diseases, Mayo Clinic College of Medicine, Rochester, Minnesota

ARTI CHOURE, MD, Department of Cardiovascular Medicine, Cleveland Clinic, Cleveland, Ohio

LORI B. DANIELS, MD, Clinical Instructor in Medicine, Division of Cardiology, University of California, San Diego, California

ADOLFO J. DE BOLD, PhD, FRCS, Professor of Pathology and Laboratory Medicine, and Cell and Molecular Medicine, Faculty of Medicine, University of Ottawa; and Director, Cardiovascular Endocrinology Laboratory, University of Ottawa Heart Institute, Ottawa, Ontario, Canada

GARY S. FRANCIS, MD, Head, Section of Clinical Cardiology, Department of Cardiovascular Medicine, Cleveland Clinic; and Professor of Medicine, Cleveland Clinic Lerner College of Medicine, Case Western Reserve University, Cleveland, Ohio

BENJAMIN J. FREDA, DO, Assistant Professor, Division of Nephrology, Tufts University School of Medicine, Baystate Medical Center, Springfield, Massachusetts

STEFAN JAMES, MD, PhD, Director of Catheterization Laboratory, Department of Cardiology and Uppsala Clinical Research Center, University Hospital of Uppsala, Uppsala, Sweden

BERTIL LINDAHL, MD, PhD, Associate Professor of Cardiology, Department of Cardiology and Uppsala Clinical Research Center, University Hospital of Uppsala, Uppsala, Sweden

ALAN S. MAISEL, MD, FACC, Professor of Medicine, University of California; Director of Coronary Care Unit and Heart Failure, Veterans Affairs Health Care System, San Diego, California

ROGER M. MILLS, MD, FACC, Vice President for Medical Affairs, Scios Inc., Fremont, California

HUGO RAMOS, MD, Adjunct Professor of Medicine, Faculty of Medicine, National University of Cordoba; and Department of Emergency Medicine, Hospital Municipal de Urgencias, Cordoba, Argentina

MARGARET M. REDFIELD, MD, Professor of Medicine, Cardiorenal Research Laboratory, Division of Cardiovascular Diseases, Mayo Clinic, Rochester, Minnesota

A. MARK RICHARDS, MD, PhD, DSc, FRACP, Department of Medicine, Christchurch School of Medicine & Health Sciences, Christchurch, New Zealand

W.H. WILSON TANG, MD, FACC, Assistant Professor of Medicine, Cleveland Clinic Lerner College of Medicine, Case Western Reserve University; Staff Cardiologist, Section of Heart Failure and Cardiac Transplantation Medicine, Department of Cardiovascular Medicine, Cleveland Clinic, Cleveland, Ohio

RICHARD W. TROUGHTON, MD, PhD, FRACP, Department of Medicine, Christchurch School of Medicine & Health Sciences, Christchurch, New Zealand

ALAN H.B. WU, PhD, Professor of Laboratory Medicine, Department of Laboratory Medicine, and Chief, Clinical Chemistry Laboratory, University of California San Francisco, San Francisco General Hospital, San Francisco, California

CLYDE W. YANCY, MD, Medical Director, Heart and Vascular Institute, Baylor University Medical Center, Dallas, Texas

CONTENTS

Editorial: Natriuretic Peptides in Heart Failure: Empathizing with the Sobbing Heart...   xi
Jagat Narula and James B. Young

Preface   xv
Roger M. Mills, W.H. Wilson Tang, and John C. Burnett, Jr

New Understanding of Natriuretic Peptides

Gene Expression, Processing, and Secretion of Natriuretic Peptides: Physiologic and Diagnostic Implications   255
Hugo Ramos and Adolfo J. de Bold

> Two polypeptide hormones—atrial natriuretic factor or peptide (ANF, ANP) and brain natriuretic peptide (BNP)—mediate the endocrine function of the heart. ANF and BNP critically modulate the activity of systems that tend to increase cardiovascular volume and pressure loads such as the rennin-angiotensin-aldosterone and sympathetic systems. Changes in hemodynamic load to the heart and in the neuroendocrine environment change the circulating levels of ANF and BNP in such a manner that the blood levels of these hormones can be used for diagnostic and prognostic purposes and to guide therapy. In addition, ANF and BNP have properties that may be beneficial in the treatment of chronic congestive heart failure and in other syndromes that are characterized by an excess pressure or volume load of the cardiovascular system. Finally, the powerful effects of cardiac natriuretic peptides on cell proliferation and growth makes them of potential benefit in cardiac remodeling.

Natriuretic Peptides as Regulators of Myocardial Structure and Function: Pathophysiologic and Therapeutic Implications   269
Alessandro Cataliotti, Horng H. Chen, Margaret M. Redfield, and John C. Burnett, Jr

> The longstanding conventional view of the natriuretic peptide system is one in which the natriuretic peptides form an important cardiorenal endocrine axis. Specifically, the heart synthesizes and releases atrial natriuretic peptide (ANP) and brain natriuretic peptide (BNP) that function to optimize intravascular volume and arterial pressure. This homeostatic function is mediated by renal, vascular, and endocrine actions that adapt to the volume status of the individual. This article diverges from this concept and advances an emerging paradigm for the natriuretic peptides as a regulator of cardiac structure

and function. Evidence suggests a deficiency of biologically active natriuretic peptides in heart failure and hypertension, arguing for the use of the natriuretic peptides as therapy to maintain optimal myocardial structure and function.

Natriuretic Peptides and Renal Insufficiency: Clinical Significance and Role of Renal Clearance 277
Benjamin J. Freda and Gary S. Francis

This article serves as a review of the role of the kidney in the metabolism and clearance of BNP and NT-proBNP. The clinical usefulness of NP testing is also discussed with attention to diagnostic performance in patients who have heart failure and concomitant renal dysfunction and patients who have various stages of chronic kidney disease being evaluated for the presence of cardiovascular disease and cardiovascular risk.

Natriuretic Peptides as Diagnostic Tests

Plasma BNP/NT-proBNP Assays: What Do They Target and What Else Might They Recognize? 291
Alan H.B. Wu

Commercial assays for B-type natriuretic peptide and the amino-terminus NT-proBNP have been cleared by the U.S. Food and Drug Administration and are now widely used biomarkers for heart failure diagnosis, staging, and risk stratification for future adverse events. Increased concentrations of BNP and NT-proBNP are also predictive for cardiovascular deaths for patients who present with acute coronary syndromes, and some commercial assays have received clearance for this indication also. In the future, results of BNP and NT-proBNP testing may be important in monitoring outpatient drug therapy of heart failure patients and for screening for left ventricular dysfunction in patients who are asymptomatic for heart failure. None of the commercial assays have clearance for these latter indications to date, however.

Natriuretic Peptides as Diagnostic Test: Lessons From the First 5 Years of Clinical Application 299
Lori B. Daniels and Alan S. Maisel

Congestive heart failure (CHF) is a growing problem in the United States but can be a difficult diagnosis to make in the acute care setting owing to the diversity of the clinical syndrome and its presentation. Over the past 5 years, natriuretic peptides have developed into a powerful aid to help clinicians with this challenging diagnosis. The use of BNP and NT-proBNP in combination with traditional diagnostic tools is enabling providers to diagnose, triage, and treat CHF patients with increasing accuracy, expediency, and efficiency. Continued clinical experience with BNP and NT-proBNP will help to further refine clinical algorithms for diagnosing, monitoring, and treating patients with heart failure, and will improve the care these patients receive.

Diagnostic Applications of Natriuretic Peptides in Ischemic Heart Disease 311
Bertil Lindahl and Stefan James

Studies of the use of the natriuretic peptides NT-proBNP and BNP for prognosis and selection of treatment selection in acute coronary syndromes and stable angina pectoris are reviewed in this article. The studies convincingly show that elevation of NT-proBNP or BNP is associated with increased mortality and that the level of NT-proBNP or BNP provides strong and independent prognostic information regardless of type of presentation of the ischemic heart disease. Although there is some evidence suggesting that measurements of NT-proBNP or BNP might be useful for selection of therapy, this important issue needs further investigation.

Natriuretic Peptides in Screening for Cardiac Dysfunction 323
W.H. Wilson Tang

> Heart failure is a devastating and costly disease. It is believed to progress in at-risk patients from a preclinical, asymptomatic stage with demonstrable heart muscle abnormalities, to an overt symptomatic heart failure syndrome. Early identification and treatment of factors that lead to myocardial dysfunction may abrogate progression to symptomatic advanced heart failure. The diagnostic usefulness of B-type natriuretic peptide (BNP) and aminoterminal-proBNP in the acute setting prompted interest in the evaluation of these clinically available biomarkers as effective screening tools. This article outlines the challenges for natriuretic peptide screening for left ventricular systolic dysfunction. In addition, it reviews the concept of optimal screening strategies based on cost-effectiveness analyses, and examines recent data regarding the usefulness of natriuretic screening for specific patient populations.

BNP for Clinical Monitoring of Heart Failure 333
Richard W. Troughton and A. Mark Richards

> Recent evidence suggests that the B-type natriuretic peptides, BNP and NT-proBNP, may be useful for monitoring and guiding optimization of therapy for heart failure (HF). Elevated plasma levels in HF reflect the severity of symptoms and cardiac dysfunction. Observational studies show that serial BNP testing identifies response to therapy, and provides incremental risk stratification over a single baseline level. BNP and NT-proBNP levels decrease with effective diuretic, vasodilator, and longer-term β-blocker therapy. Plasma levels also may identify patients who are most likely to benefit from medical therapy. Recent studies suggest that titrating medical therapy to achieve BNP or NT-proBNP levels below a target range may improve clinical outcomes compared with empiric strategies. The results of larger randomized studies testing the efficacy of BNP or NT-proBNP guided pharmacotherapy for heart failure are keenly awaited.

Natriuretic Peptides in Valvular Heart Diseases 345
Arti Choure, W.H. Wilson Tang, and Roger M. Mills

> Natriuretic peptide testing has been proposed as a marker of disease severity in valvular heart diseases, especially in patients who have poor echocardiographic windows. This inexpensive blood test may provide the opportunity to monitor disease progression between echocardiographic testing intervals. Data regarding the use of these biomarkers in the setting of valvular heart diseases have been limited, however. This article reviews the published literature evaluating the role of natriuretic peptide levels in the evaluation and management of left-sided valvular heart diseases and attempts to synthesize the findings into pragmatic recommendations.

Natriuretic Peptides as Therapeutic Agents

B-Type Natriuretic Peptides in Management of Acute Decompensated Heart Failure 353
Clyde W. Yancy

> Acute decompensated heart failure (ADHF) is a compelling complication of heart failure. There is an incomplete understanding of its pathophysiology, and minimally effective treatment options exist. Currently, treatment is targeted toward abnormal hemodynamics and includes diuretics, vasodilators, and inotropes. B-type natriuretic peptide represents a novel therapeutic option for ADHF that lowers elevated filling pressures and improves dyspnea. The risk-benefit ratio remains an unresolved issue because questions persist regarding drug-related morbidity and mortality. More research is needed to identify the ideal clinical scenario and to resolve the absence or presence of drug-associated risks.

Therapeutic Potential for Existing and Novel Forms of Natriuretic Peptides 365
Horng H. Chen and John C. Burnett Jr

The natriuretic peptides are a family of peptides, each with a 17—amino acid disulfide ring structure, that are genetically distinct with diverse actions in cardiovascular, renal, and endocrine homeostasis. In humans, the family consists of atrial natriuretic peptide (ANP) and brain natriuretic peptide (BNP) of myocardial cell origin, C-type natriuretic peptide (CNP) of endothelial origin, and urodilatin (Uro) thought to be derived from the kidney. This review provides an update on important issues regarding the therapeutic potential of existing and novel forms of natriuretic peptides beyond acute decompensated heart failure.

Index 375

FORTHCOMING ISSUES

October 2006
Valvular Disease and Heart Failure
Blasé Anthony Carabello, MD, *Guest Editor*

January 2007
Advances in Heart Transplantation
Mandeep R. Mehra, MD, *Guest Editor*

April 2007
The Role of Surgery
Stephen Westaby, BSc, MS, PhD,
and Mario C. Deng, MD, *Guest Editors*

RECENT ISSUES

April 2006
Noninvasive Imaging of Heart Failure
Vasken Dilsizian, MD, Mario J. Garcia, MD,
and David Bello, MD, *Guest Editors*

January 2006
Diabetic-Hypertensive Pre–Heart Failure Patient
David S.H. Bell, MB, *Guest Editor*

October 2005
Myocarditis
G. William Dec, MD, *Guest Editor*

THE CLINICS ARE NOW AVAILABLE ONLINE!

Access your subscription at:
http://www.theclinics.com

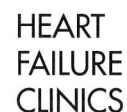

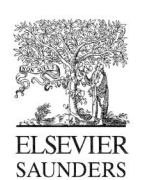

Editorial

Natriuretic Peptides in Heart Failure: Empathizing with the Sobbing Heart...

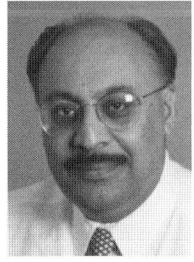

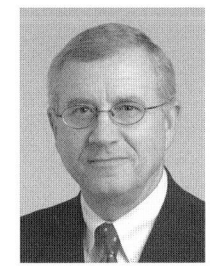

Jagat Narula, MD, PhD   James B. Young, MD
Consulting Editors

Over the last five years, we have witnessed a meteoric rise in the use of measuring B-type natriuetic peptide (BNP) as a biomarker in cardiovascular disease. Although initially its use was proposed as a simple diagnostic tool to aid in the clinical assessment of decompensated heart failure, studies have now shown that BNP perturbation is, more generally, a marker of myocardial stress and offers enormous diagnostic as well as prognostic information in a variety of settings, including cardiomyopathy, congestive heart failure syndromes, ischemic heart disease, and even pulmonary thrombo-embolism. Decompensated heart failure patients with very high levels of BNP who do not substantially improve prior to hospital discharge are at a high risk of readmission or death in a very short time. Furthermore, the higher the BNP level in patients with acute coronary syndromes, the worse the prognosis, and this observation actually supplements information based on troponin levels, coronary anatomy, and left ventricular function. We also now know that an increase in BNP level occurs with development of manifest myocardial ischemia during exercise. Also important is the observation that even in the "high normal" BNP level range, despite the absence of symptoms, the general population will have a higher likelihood of major cardiovascular events over time, including development of symptomatic heart failure.

Although A-type natriuretic peptide (ANP) has long been tried as a therapeutic agent in patients with decompensated heart failure, introduction of the genetically engineered BNP has been extremely promising for the management of heart failure. Use of intravenously administered BNP in these individuals has been shown to decrease symptoms, reduce length of hospital stay, improve short-term mortality, and optimize patient management. Although some controversy has recently surfaced regarding mortality in patients with compromised renal function receiving BNP, results from larger and creatively designed randomized clinical trials are awaited for the final verdict. Most observers believe, however, that in appropriately selected and treated individuals, mortality and morbidity is reduced with BNP therapy.

It is intriguing that even though the levels of natriuretic peptides are significantly higher in heart failure patients than in normal individuals or those

1551-7136/06/$ - see front matter © 2006 Elsevier Inc. All rights reserved.
doi:10.1016/j.hfc.2006.09.004

heartfailure.theclinics.com

with clinically compensated ventricular dysfunction, infusion of exogenous BNP is effective! The evolution of natriuretic peptides may offer some explanation for this seeming paradox. The family of natriuretic peptides has grown as species have evolved, and its role has become increasingly important in organism homeostasis, with respect to intra- and extravascular volume control and osmotic and barometric loading of the circulatory system. This increasing role of natriuretic peptides through time was probably in response to the requirements of aquatic life. Although some form of natriuretic peptide can be traced to lower invertebrates and plants, the true evolution started around 550 million years ago, in elasmobranchs, such as the shark (Fig. 1). The C-type natriuretic peptide (CNP) seems to be the ancestral peptide. Elegant studies [1,2] have proposed that at that time, four CNP genes (CNP1–4) developed by chromosomal duplication. Of the initial CNP3 and -4 genes, CNP3 persisted up to amphibians and was subsequently lost. However, it diversified into the ANP and BNP genes before teleosts originated. CNP4 is retained in humans as CNP. On the other hand, the CNP1 and -2 genes evolved before teleosts but were immediately lost in tetrapods.

It is interesting to note that the need for natriuretic peptides has dwindled since the divergence of the amphibians. Aquatic and marine animals required aquauretic and natriuretic systems for survival. As life became terrestrial, animals began to require salt and water conservation (a transition from a state of salt excess to a state of sodium deficiency) [3,4]. Sodium deficiency is an ecological stress, and the study of comparative endocrinology reveals that the secretion of aldosterone emerged at an early stage of vertebrate evolution, facilitating electrolyte regulation in special tissues. Sharks have a glomerular kidney but no renin-angiotensin system. At a later stage in phylogenetic development (the amphibian and terrestrial life forms), additional mechanisms of humoral stimulation of aldosterone secretion emerged, with an added function of supporting systemic blood pressure—the renin-angiotensin system. The renin–angiotensin axis bloomed and matured in mammals. We can surmise that the natriuretic peptides have been reduced to vestigial hormones in terrestrial animals [3,4]. This notion is based on the fact that the increase in the effective levels of natriuretic peptides, at least ANP, does not exceed 500 pg/mL, which is lower than the minimum pharmacologically effective dose (equivalent to a plasma level of 600 pg/mL). In the case of BNP, it seems that although the hormone may be produced in enormously large quantities, either the processing of prohormones to active fragments is inadequate or the

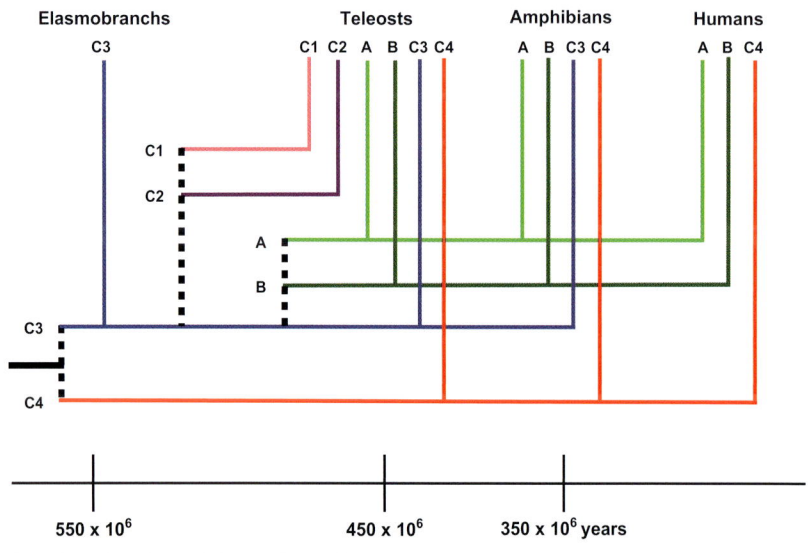

Fig. 1. Evolution of natriuretic peptides. (*Adapted from* Inoue K, Naruse K, Yamagami S, et al. Four functionally distinct C-type natriuretic peptides found in fish reveal evolutionary history of natriuretic peptides. Proc Natl Acad Sci USA 2003;100:10079–84.)

mediators of signal transduction are markedly deficient. Although the production of natriuretic peptides in heart failure seems to be a manifestation of the fetal phenotype (or phylogenetic reversal), the capability of the myocardium to efficiently produce and process natriuretic peptides remains markedly limited. Clearly, we have much to learn about the important and fascinating regulatory–counter regulatory cardiovascular hormones as diagnostic, prognostic, and therapeutic agents.

It is as though the myocardium sheds a stream of tears into the ventricular cavity when in distress. Although the tears may not control the pain, they do tell of its extent!

Jagat Narula, MD, PhD
Professor, Medicine
Chief, Division of Cardiology
Associate Dean
University of California
School of Medicine
101 The City Drive
Building 53, Mail Route 81
Irvine, CA 92868-4080, USA

E-mail address: narula@uci.edu

James B. Young, MD
Chairman, Department of Medicine
Professor, Medicine
Lerner College of Medicine
Case Western Reserve University
Cleveland Clinic Foundation
9500 Euclid Avenue
Desk T-13
Cleveland, OH 44195, USA

E-mail address: youngj@ccf.org

References

[1] Inoue K, Naruse K, Yamagami S, et al. Four functionally distinct C-type natriuretic peptides found in fish reveal evolutionary history of the natriuretic peptide system. Proc Natl Acad Sci USA 2003;100: 10079–84.
[2] Takei Y. Does the natriuretic peptide system exist throughout the animal and plant kingdom?. Comp Biochem Physiol B Biochem Mol Biol 2001;129: 559–73.
[3] Vasan RS, Seshadri S, Narula J. Atrial natriuretic peptide: an atavistic hormone?. Int J Cardiol 1989; 24:404–5.
[4] Vasan RS, Seshadri S, Narula J. Atrial natriuretic peptide: action yes, role no!. Int J Cardiol 1989;25: 142–3.

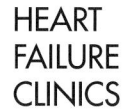

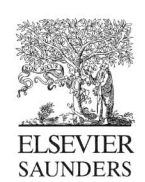

Preface

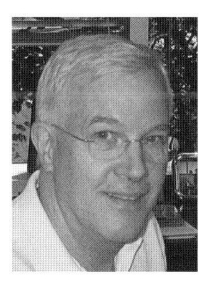

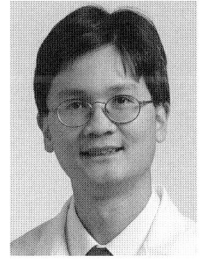

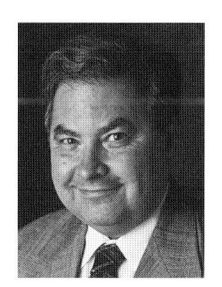

Roger M. Mills, MD   W.H. Wilson Tang, MD   John C. Burnett, Jr, MD
Guest Editors

This issue marks the 25th anniversary of the discovery of the natriuretic peptide system by Professor de Bold [1]. The 11 articles in this issue that focus on natriuretic peptides differ substantially from many review compilations. In the articles to follow, readers will find a wealth of authoritative, well-documented, and informative discussions. As editors, we are proud that many of our authors are world leaders in their respective fields; many of them have made substantial contributions to our contemporary understanding of the natriuretic peptide system. However, most of the articles will raise more questions than they answer, and our goal in this preface is to put those questions in context.

In 1967, Braunwald, Ross, and Sonnenblick [2] reached the summit in the long trek to describe the mechanics of cardiac function with the publication of their multi-part review, "Mechanisms of contraction of the normal and failing heart," in the New England Journal of Medicine. In the 40 years since that landmark publication, cardiovascular researchers and clinicians have come to realize that cardiovascular physiology and pathophysiology are intimately interwoven with the physiology of salt and water regulation. Our task now is the integration of neuroendocrine, renal, and cardiovascular data to better understand normal physiology and to better manage patients with cardiovascular disease with therapeutic manipulations.

Since early aquatic vertebrates first exploited a favorable ecologic niche with the strategy of reproducing in fresh water and maturing in salt water, vertebrate physiology has developed highly conserved systems to retain and to eliminate salt and water: the rennin-angiotensin-aldosterone and natriuretic peptide systems. This issue is an update on the journey toward understanding how the natriuretic peptide system functions in health and disease, acutely and chronically, impacting the brain, the heart, and the kidney. Many of the authors represent research laboratories that have brought us pivotal insights into natriuretic peptide biology, as well as relevant clinical applications in the diagnosis and therapy of heart failure. It is not a journal of a trip completed, as "mechanisms of contraction" was, but a collection of reports from experts exploring the many different routes that have led to our current understanding of the role of the natriuretic peptide system.

Finally, the editors and authors would like to acknowledge Karen Sorensen, Senior Clinics Editor at Elsevier, for her assistance and, most of all, for her patience with the writing of this issue.

Roger M. Mills, MD
Scios, Inc.
6500 Paseo Padre Parkway
Fremont, CA 94555 USA

E-mail address: rmills@scius.jnj.com

W.H. Wilson Tang, MD
Department of Cardiovascular Medicine
The Cleveland Clinic
9500 Euclid Avenue, Desk F25
Cleveland, OH 44195 USA

E-mail address: tangw@ccf.org

John C. Burnett, Jr, MD
Cardiorenal Research Laboratory
Department of Cardiovascular Diseases
Mayo Clinic
200 First Street SW
Rochester, MN 55905 USA

E-mail address: Burnett.john@mayo.edu

References

[1] de Bold AJ, Borenstein HB, Veress AT, et al. A rapid and potent natriuretic response to intravenous injection of atrial myocardial extract in rats. Life Sci 1981;28(1):89–94.

[2] Braunwald E, Ross J Jr, Sonnenblick EH. Mechanisms of contraction of the normal and failing heart. N Engl J Med 1967;277:794–800, 853–63, 910–20, 962–71, 1012–22.

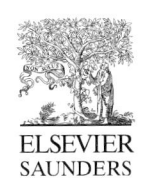

Gene Expression, Processing, and Secretion of Natriuretic Peptides: Physiologic and Diagnostic Implications

Hugo Ramos, MD[a], Adolfo J. de Bold, PhD, FRCS[b],*

[a]*Hospital de Urgencias, National University of Cordoba, Córdoba, Argentina*
[b]*University of Ottawa Heart Institute, Ottawa, ON, Canada*

The cardiac natriuretic peptide (NP) system is composed of atrial natriuretic factor (ANF) [1,2] and brain natriuretic peptide (BNP) [3]. These polypeptide hormones are synthesized, stored, and secreted by cardiocytes in the atria of the mammalian heart (Fig. 1). ANF and BNP are co-stored in storage granules that are referred to as specific atrial granules. Under normal circumstances, small amounts of ANF and BNP also are synthesized by the normal ventricular cardiocytes and in several noncardiac sites (eg, central nervous system, gonads, kidneys). NP can modulate the activity of intrinsic renal mechanisms, the sympathetic nervous system, the renin-angiotensin-aldosterone system, and other determinants of vascular tone and renal function [3]. Because of these properties, the NPs limit increases in extracellular fluid volume and blood pressure. In addition, the NPs have potent growth-regulating properties, which make them of interest in the regulation of cardiovascular growth, including cardiac remodeling following an acute myocardial infarction and congestive heart failure. NPs signal mainly through increases in cGMP in target cells following activation of guanylyl cyclase-coupled receptors. ANF and BNP are agonists of the type A NP receptor (NPRA). Intracellular cGMP receptors include cGMP-dependent protein kinases, cGMP-gated ion channels, and cGMP-regulated cyclic nucleotide phosphodiesterases [4].

Attesting to the pathophysiologic and physiologic importance of the NP system, investigations showed that pharmacologic blockade of the NP receptor or genetic disruption of NP genes or their receptors results in impairment of cardiorenal homeostasis [5–7]. Genetic knockout of the ANF or the NPRA genes leads to salt-sensitive or salt-insensitive hypertension, respectively, in homozygous null mice [8,9]. In NPRA-deficient homozygous mice, volume expansion fails to induce diuresis and natriuresis and to increase cGMP excretion as observed in wild-type mice that were treated identically [9]. In another NPRA knockout model, absence of NPRA causes hypertension and leads to cardiac hypertrophy with extensive interstitial fibrosis and, particularly in males, to sudden death [10]. BNP knockouts do not develop hypertension or cardiac hypertrophy, but do show cardiac fibrosis [11].

Genetic expression of cardiac natriuretic peptides

The secretory-like morphologic differentiations that are associated with the endocrine function of the heart and NP, which in adult mammals mainly are restricted to cardiocytes of the atrial chambers (Fig. 2), find their counterparts in atrial and ventricular cardiocytes in nonmammalian vertebrates, such as aves, amphibians, and teleost fishes, as well as in several nonvertebrate species (eg, shark). Beyond the cellular phenotype, there are significant differences between species at the molecular level in the type and relative

---

* Corresponding author. Cardiovascular Endocrinology Laboratory, University of Ottawa Heart Institute, 40 Ruskin Street, Ottawa, ON K1Y 4W7, Canada.
   E-mail address: adebold@ottawaheart.ca
(A.J. de Bold).

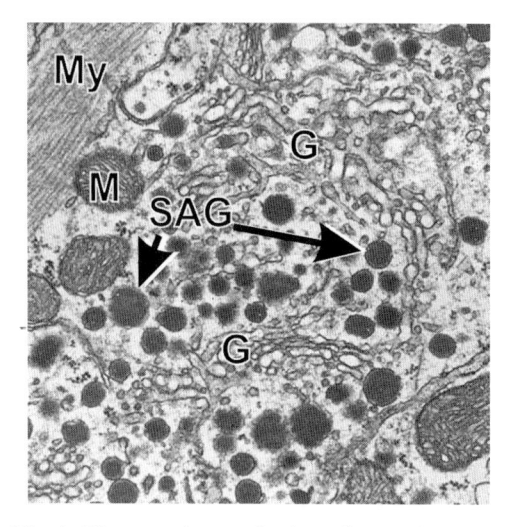

Fig. 1. Electron microscopic view of a portion of an atrial cardiocyte showing the specific atrial granules (SAG), Golgi complex (G), mitochondria (M), and myofibrils (My).

level of expression of the NPs and their receptors [12–15].

During heart development, ANF is an early marker for the formation of the working myocardium of atrial and ventricular chambers. Shortly after birth the expression of the ANF and BNP genes is silenced in ventricular cardiocytes. The tissue specificity and spatiotemporal expression of genes (eg, the NP genes) are governed by specific DNA sequences (cis-acting sequences) that are found in the promoter portion of the NP genes. The expression of a given gene, including those that encode NP, under physiologic or pathophysiologic conditions can be up-regulated or down-regulated through this mechanism [16–50].

The specific NP mRNAs are abundant in the atria, and account for about 2% of total RNA. Other sites, such as the ventricles and portions of the ventricular-conducting system, express ANF and BNP, albeit at much lower levels than in the atria [51].

Processing of cardiac natriuretic peptides

In atrial cardiocytes, newly synthesized ANF and BNP follow vectorial transport from their site of synthesis in the endoplasmic reticulum to the Golgi complex where they are packaged together and concentrated into the specific atrial secretory granules (Fig. 3). The human prohormones that arise from processing of the ANF and BNP preprohormones are ANF_{1-126} and BNP_{1-108}. ANF is stored in the atrial granules as the precursor form $proANF_{1-126}$, whereas BNP is stored as the C-terminal portion (CT-BNP) BNP_{77-108}, which is its circulating form [52,53]. During the secretory process, proANF is processed further to the circulating C-terminal portion, bioactive form ANF_{99-126} (CT-ANF). The N-terminal portions of the ANF (NT-ANF) and BNP (NT-BNP) prohormones also circulate in blood in a manner that reflects the secretory state of the bioactive ANF and BNP hormones; a fact that has been taken advantage of in the development of clinical laboratory measurements of the activity of the cardiac NP system.

Secretion of cardiac natriuretic peptides

Basal secretion

ANF and BNP are secreted with identical kinetics from the atria as would be expected for hormones that are stored in the same granule. These hormones are secreted continuously, even in the absence of discernible stimuli in vivo or in vitro. This baseline secretion is insensitive to the protein synthesis inhibitor cycloheximide [54]. Additional characteristics of the basal secretory process of atrial NP are that removal of Ca^{+2} from the perfusion media in the isolated atrial preparation results, contrary to expectation for a polypeptide hormone–producing tissue, in a significant increase in ANF secretion. In this sense, atrial secretory function is similar to that observed for renin secretion from juxtaglomerular cells [55,56]. In vitro, a stepwise increase in pacing frequency of the left atrium from 0.2 to 2.0 Hz results in a significant decrease in ANF secretion [57]. These observations have been confirmed using perfused rat hearts [58] and rabbit atria [59]. Finally, depolarization with medium that contains high K^+ (49 mM) does not affect ANF secretion [60]. The authors have concluded that although indispensable for excitation-contraction coupling, intracellular Ca^{2+} transients by influx or from intracellular stores are not essential for basal ANF release.

Stimulated secretion

Appropriate changes in the hemodynamic and neurohumoral environments can increase the rate of NP secretion significantly. Investigations using monensin, an ionophore that impairs protein sorting and transport in the trans-Golgi network and inhibits vesicle formation, as well as double pulse-chase experiments using

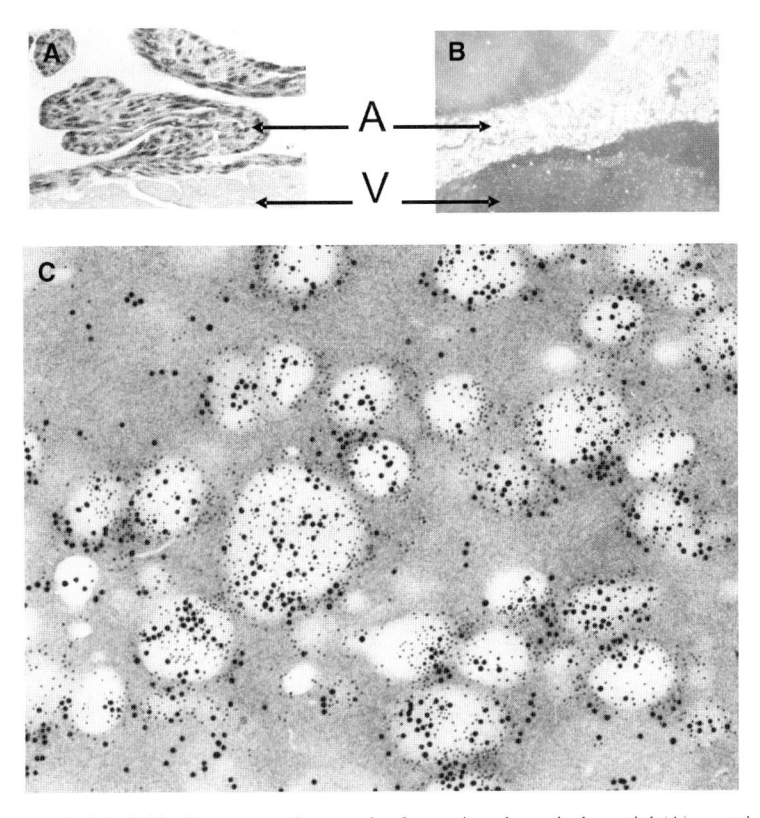

Fig. 2. (A) Low-power bright-field microscopy micrograph of a section through the atrial (A)–ventricular (V) junction showing ANF immunoreactivity in atrial cardiocytes. (B) ANF mRNA by in situ hybridization signal photographed using dark-field microscopy. Technical details are published elsewhere [106,107]. (C) High-power electron microscopic photograph of atrial specific granules, which appear as negative images, showing colocalization of ANF (smaller gold particles) and BNP (larger gold particles).

^{3}H-leucine to label ANF, show that the bulk of the stimulated response of the atria is based on newly formed secretory granules. Furthermore, although monensin totally abrogated the stimulated response it did not affect baseline release [54,61]. Overall, these findings show that NP secretion from the atria is based on a pool of newly synthesized hormone that is released promptly, while a portion of the hormone proceeds to a storage pool from where it is released slowly. This is reminiscent of the constitutive-like secretory pathway that has been observed in the pancreas where secretion is based on the exocytosis of vesicles that bud from immature granules [62–64].

Two main types of stimuli that promote NP secretion generally are recognized. One such type is related to the increase in NP secretion that is observed upon muscle stretch, whereas the second type is related to the stimulation of NP secretion by hormones that signal through G-protein–coupled receptors, such as endothelin-1 (ET-1). Two distinguishing features between these types are the kinetics of secretion following stimulation [60] (virtually instantaneous for stretch as compared with a slower onset for hormonally mediated stimulation) and the sensitivity to Pertussis toxin, which abrogates the stretch-stimulated secretion [65].

The increased secretion of ANF following mechanical stretch is referred to as stretch-secretion coupling [60]. Following muscle stretch, ANF is released from a depletable pool of newly formed granules in a manner that is characterized by a phasic, short-term (ie, minutes) burst of NP secretion, independently of NP synthesis [66]. The acute secretion of NPs that is observed during head-out water immersion is based on stretch-secretion coupling [67,68], which arises from the induction of increased central venous return and

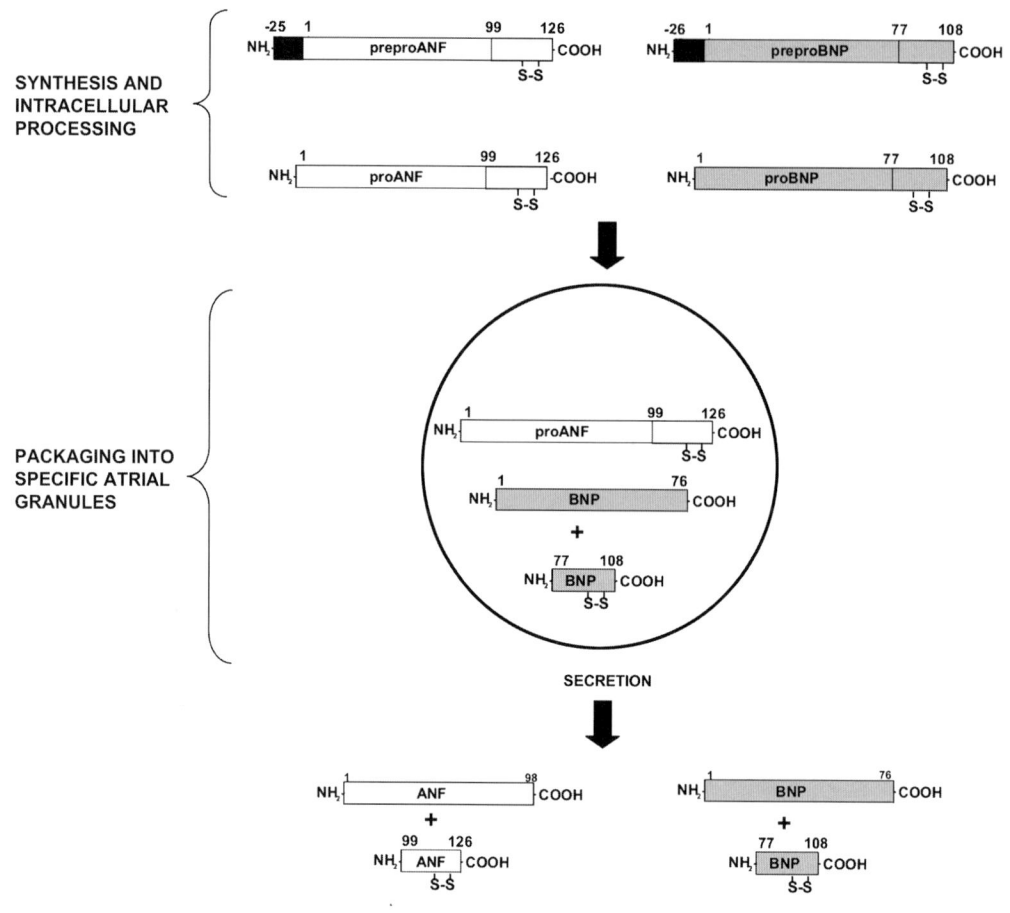

Fig. 3. Processing of cardiac NP precursors in atrial cardiocytes giving rise to the N-terminal and C-terminal portions of the ANF and BNP prohormones. The tissue concentration ratio of ANF/BNP in atrial tissue is approximately 100:1 to 1000:1.

ensuing atrial stretch. It is stretch, and not pressure, that causes increased secretion of NP as shown in humans who have cardiac tamponade in whom increased atrial pressure with no atrial stretch does not result in increased ANF circulating levels. Thus, increased atrial stretch, rather than atrial pressure, is the key stimulus for acute ANF secretion [69–71].

Neurohumors and other substances, such as ET-1 [72], hydroxyvitamin D3 [73], glucocorticoids, thyroid hormone, growth factors, thrombin, angiotensin II, prostaglandins, and α_1-adrenergic agonists [69], promote NP secretion, and, often, genetic expression of NPs in vitro in the absence of mechanical stimulation. Some of these substances contribute actively to the modulation of ANF and BNP synthesis and secretion in the normal and pathophysiologic states, where a combination of hemodynamic and neurohumoral stimuli coexist [74,75].

A special subacute type of stimulated NP secretion is observed during mineralocorticoid escape. Chronic administration of mineralocorticoid in vivo results in a period of positive sodium balance followed by a brisk natriuresis when the kidney "escapes" the salt-retaining effect of the mineralocorticoid. The increase in intravascular volume that ensues from mineralocorticoid administration leads to increased NP gene expression and secretion by the atria. The authors showed that in vivo blockade of the NP receptor by the compound HS-142-1 significantly reduces that ability of the kidney to effect a mineralocorticoid escape [7]. The increase in NP gene expression that is observed during mineralocorticoid escape is restricted to the atria.

Under chronic hemodynamic overload conditions, as seen in long-standing hypertension and in chronic congestive heart failure, ventricular cardiocytes undergo dramatic phenotypical alterations, which are accompanied by a partial re-expression of cardiac genes that encode for proteins that usually are present in fetal life. Included in these proteins are ANF and BNP and the fetal isoform of myosin heavy chain. For unknown reasons, although ANF and BNP also are up-regulated in the atria under these conditions, the myosin heavy chain isoform switch does not occur.

Hemodynamic and neurohumoral determinants of cardiac natriuretic peptide gene expression

In an attempt to assess the separate contributions of hemodynamic load and of neuroendocrine changes to the expression and secretion of cardiac NP, the authors used rats with experimentally induced renovascular hypertension that were treated with dosage schedules of the angiotensin-converting enzyme (ACE) inhibitor Ramipril resulted in the prevention or regression of hypertension and hypertrophy (high dosage) or in the regression of hypertrophy alone with persistent hypertension (low dosage). They demonstrated that NP production and secretion are related independently to increased blood pressure and hypertrophy. That is, regression of ventricular hypertrophy in the presence of hypertension decreases circulating levels of NP only partially, although this regression is accompanied by normalization of ventricular NP gene expression [76].

Further insight into the regulation of NP gene expression in the heart in pathophysiologic conditions may be gleaned from experiments in which an endothelin type A receptor antagonist was administered to deoxycorticosterone acetate (DOCA) salt or Goldblatt hypertensive rats with left ventricular hypertrophy. Treatment with the endothelin antagonist normalized ventricular NP gene expression but did not affect atrial NP gene expression. This suggested that there are significant differences in the mechanisms that control NP production between atrial and ventricular cardiocytes; the latter seems to be dependent on humoral factors to a significant degree, but certainly not on wall tension alone [75,77].

Qualitatively, the relative expression of atrial and ventricular NPs is similar in normal and pathophysiologic circumstances. In the normal rat heart, for example, the left atrial content of CT-ANF and CT-BNP are 30,000 and 300 pmol/g, respectively, whereas left ventricular CT-ANF and CT-BNP content are 5 and 1.5 pmol/g, respectively. In the hypertrophic left ventricle the amounts of CT-ANF and CT-BNP increase to 70 and 5 pmol/g, respectively [53]. These values are contrary to the notion that views ANF as an atrial hormone and BNP as a ventricular hormone.

Highest levels of circulating ANF and BNP are found in patients who have advanced heart failure. Blood samples from patients who were in end-stage heart failure before transplantation had CT-ANF and CT-BNP plasma levels (mean ± SEM) of 356 ± 21 pg/mL (n = 77) and 259 ± 37 pg/mL (n = 76), respectively (authors' unpublished data). Replacement of the failing ventricle—as is done in orthotopic heart transplantation—does not result in normalization of BNP or ANF plasma levels, even after normalization of intracardiac pressures and the renin-angiotensin-aldosterone system occurs [78–80]. Lastly, cardiac catheterization data in humans who have left ventricular hypertrophy suggest that the abnormal circulating levels of NP are derived significantly from atrial sources [81]. These findings show that although there may be a good correlation between ventricular function and NP secretion, the influence of these parameters on atrial function, and, hence, on atrial NP production, should not be ignored. Moreover, the combined data do not support the view that BNP should be viewed solely as a ventricular hormone, although the relative increase of BNP in certain pathologic conditions that affect the heart is larger than is the increase of ANF. This happens without changing the concept that ANF concentration in atria, ventricles, and blood is larger than that of BNP under most circumstances. An interesting and potentially important exception is that observed in acute cardiac allograft rejection [79,80], in in vitro studies that used cultured ventricular cardiocytes that were exposed to proinflammatory cytokines [39], and in experimentally induced autoimmune myocarditis (unpublished data). Under all of these circumstances, BNP, and not ANF, is up-regulated. These are the only known instances of exclusive up-regulation of an NP seemingly having an inflammation component in common.

Natriuretic peptides and cardiovascular disease

Soon after the development of specific and sensitive radioimmunoassay (RIAs) for ANF in plasma, it was apparent that the circulating levels of this hormone were elevated significantly in

Table 1
Natriuretic peptides in acute coronary syndromes

Study	n	Type of ACS	Biomarker	Initial sampling time or median	Follow-up	Main findings
Fontana et al [108]	16	AMI	ANF	<3 h	15 d	Significant correlation of ANF plasma values with LVEF
Ngo et al [109]	17	AMI	ANF$_{1-98}$ ANF$_{31-67}$ ANF$_{99-126}$	Presentation	14 d	NT-proANF correlated with CPK levels but not with LVEF. Unstable angina with chest pain not associated with increased NP plasma levels.
Motwani et al [85]	16	Q wave AMI	ANF BNP	2nd day	6 mo	BNP levels identify patients who would benefit from ACE inhibition.
Morita et al [110]	50	STE-AMI	ANF BNP	3.7 h	4 wk	Description of monophasic and biphasic elevation of NP post AMI.
Horio et al [111]	16	STE-AMI	ANF BNP	First 24 h	4 wk	Correlation of ANF with PWP and CI. BNP inversely correlated with LVEF.
Hall et al [84]	76	STE-AMI	NT-proANF	<4 h	1 y	NT-proANF plasma levels within 12 h after AMI a prognostic indicator of mortality at 1 y
Jernberg et al [103]	104	Unstable angina non-STE AMI	NT-proANF	<72 h	48 mo	NT-proANF was prognostic indicator related to mortality
Omland et al [112]	53	Unstable angina non-STE AMI	NT-proANF NT-proBNP	<12 h	43 d	NT-proBNP was an additional indicator to troponin I. Elevated NT-proANP and NT-proBNP plasma levels associated with early death.
de Lemos et al (OPUS-TIMI 16) [98]	2525	STE-AMI (n = 825) non-ST AMI (n = 565) Unstable angina (n = 1133)	BNP	40 h	10 mo	Defines cut-offs for prediction of death or new cardiac events and as an independent predictor of long-term risk.
Omland et al [102]	609	STE-AMI (n = 204) non-STE AMI (n = 220) Unstable angina (n = 185)	NT-proBNP	3 d	51 mo	Defines cut-off points for survivors and nonsurvivors. Gives indicator values for long-term mortality after adjustment for clinical parameters and LVEF.
James et al GUSTO IV [100]	6809	non-STE AMI Unstable angina	NT-proBNP	9.5 h	12 mo	Identifies quartiles related with short- and long-term mortality. Shows relationship to TnT and mortality and identifies a subgroup of patients at lesser risk, independently of other indicators.

Study	N	Population	Peptide	Sampling time	Follow-up	Main findings
Jernberg et al (FRISC II) [113]	2019	non-STE AMI Unstable angina	NT-proBNP	39 h	24 mo	Identifies a relationship with IL-6 plasma levels and benefit associated with early intervention
Morrow et al (TACTIS-TIMI 18) [101]	1676	non-STE AMI Unstable angina	BNP	—	6 mo	Defines cut-off points predicting death and heart failure. Shows differences in predictive value with TnT.
Galvani et al [114]	1756	non-STE AMI or STE-AMI	NT-proBNP	Median = 3 h	30 d	Validates NT-proBNP for early risk stratification
Galvani et al [104]	12474	Meta-analysis of Refs. [100,102, 114–116]	BNP/NT-proBNP	At presentation or later	-	Short- and long-term prognostic value for non-STE AMI or STE-AMI
Heeschen et al (PRISM) [115]	1401	non-STE ACS	NT-proBNP	Baseline and serial: 48 h 72 h	30 d	Levels > 250 ng/L are independent predictors of risk even with negative TnT. Serial determinations increase the predictive value compared with a single determination combined with TnT and CRP.
Lindahl et al (FRISC II) [116]	1216	non-STE ACS	NT-proBNP	Baseline and serial: 48 h 6 wk 3 and 6 mo	2 y	Measurements in the relatively stable chronic phase are better predictors of long-term mortality than are those made in the acute phase
Morrow et al (A to Z) [117]	4266	ACS	BNP	Baseline and serial: 4 and 12 mo	2 y	Levels of > 80 pg/mL at presentation or follow-up are associated with death or new heart failure
Bjorklund et al (ASSENT 2 and ASSENT PLUS) [118]	782	STE-AMI	NT-proBNP	On admission	1 y	At admission, gives together with 50% ST resolution at 60 min, important prognostic information even after adjustment for TnT and baseline characteristics in STE-AMI
James et al (GUSTO IV) [119]	7800	Non-ST ACS	NT-proBNP	9.5 h	1 y	Mean levels of NT-proBNP were twofold higher in diabetic patients. ST depression of > 0.5 mm NT-proNP > 669 ng/L, and IL-6 > 10 ng/L predicted mortality in diabetic and nondiabetic patients.

Abbreviations: AMI, acute myocardial infarction; CI, cardiac index; CPK, creatine phosphokinase; CRP, C-creative protein; IL-6, interleukin-6; LVEF, left ventricle ejection fraction; non-STE AMI, AMI without ST-segment elevation; NT, N-terminus; PWP, pulmonary wedge pressure; STE-AMI, AMI with ST-segment elevation; TnT, troponin T.

a variety of clinical conditions, all of which were underlain by an increase in pressure or volume load on the heart [82,83]. It was further established that the plasma levels of CT-ANF were, in general, proportional to the degree and duration of this overload. Thus, the highest circulating plasma CT-ANF levels were associated with long-standing essential hypertension and chronic congestive heart failure classes III and IV. Obviously, in these situations not only are hemodynamic parameters altered, but so is the neuroendocrine balance, which undoubtedly contributes to the determination of NP plasma levels. A similar historical development may be found for BNP; the development of a RIA demonstrated that elevated levels of circulating CT-BNP were an indication of long-standing pressure or volume overload. Further, in the case of BNP, a strong induction of the gene expression for these peptides was observed in the hypertrophied ventricle that resulted in a larger elevation of plasma BNP levels compared with those of ANF, although, in absolute terms, the circulating levels of ANF remained greater than those of BNP.

Having established that important clinical entities are accompanied by changes in ANF and BNP gene expression, several clinical investigators explored the possibility that ANF and BNP plasma levels may be used as diagnostic or prognostic indicators of cardiovascular disease. Earlier studies included the use of CT-ANF plasma levels to establish long-term prognosis after myocardial infarction (MI) [84], to stratify patients in terms of response to ACE inhibition after MI [85], and to demonstrate asymptomatic left ventricular dysfunction [86,87]. Richards and colleagues [88] found a good correlation between plasma CT-ANF and cardiac output in elderly patients, and showed that plasma CT-ANF was a prognostic indicator of the subsequent development of chronic heart failure. Similarly, Davis and colleagues [89] showed that in the elderly, CT-ANF plasma levels identified subjects who were at risk for congestive heart failure; this allowed for appropriate focusing of medical resources for the prevention, early detection, and treatment of this syndrome. Lerman and colleagues [86] showed that NT-ANF is a highly sensitive marker for symptomless left ventricular dysfunction. Motwani and colleagues [85] showed that BNP_{77-108} plasma levels identify patients who have left ventricular dysfunction who have been identified by the Survival and Ventricular Enlargement (SAVE) study as likely to benefit from long-term ACE inhibitor treatment after MI. In this study, plasma CT-ANF was not as predictive as was CT-BNP. The usefulness of NT-ANF plasma levels to evaluate clinical status was re-emphasized in a study by Dickstein and colleagues [90]. They showed that NT-ANF correlated better than did other variables with New York Heart Association (NYHA) functional class and was associated more closely with noninvasive measurements than with NYHA functional class. Odds ratio measurements demonstrated substantially increased risk for left ventricular dysfunction and dilatation, pulmonary hypertension, and NYHA functional class 3 or 4 with increasing NT-ANF value. The investigators concluded that the data clearly indicated that the concentration of proANF is related to the degree of clinical heart failure. Moe and colleagues [91] used NT-ANF to characterize hormonal activation in patients who had severe heart failure and were treated with flosequinan; a significant decline in plasma NT-ANF levels was observed in the survivors only. The importance of NP plasma level measurement was re-emphasized by Hall and colleagues [84]. Reporting for the Thrombolysis in Myocardial Infarction II investigators, they showed that NT-ANF, when measured during the first 12 hours after the onset of chest pain, is related to 1-year mortality after MI.

In evaluating the early literature on the use of NPs as diagnostic biomarkers and predictors of disease and on the relative merits of ANF or BNP peptide measurements, it must be kept in mind that many of the early studies used nonstandardized procedures.

Of late, much of the attention that has been directed toward the clinical measurement of NPs in blood has been focused on CT- and NT-BNP. Some of this interest is based on the fact that commercial companies have put tests—in a reproducible clinical kit format—in the hands of researchers. Maisel and colleagues evaluated the usefulness of rapid BNP test measurements [92–97]. They concluded that these tests are excellent screening tools for left ventricular systolic or diastolic dysfunction, and may preclude the need for echocardiography in many patients. The prognostic value of BNP in acute coronary syndromes was demonstrated by de Lemos and colleagues [98]. They concluded that a single measurement of BNP within a few days of the onset of ischemic symptoms predicts and risk stratifies across the spectrum of acute coronary syndromes, including MI with and without ST-segment elevation and unstable angina. Talwar and colleagues [99] examined the optimum time of blood sampling for NT-BNP determination following MI. Because they found a biphasic pattern, they concluded that NT-BNP plasma level was a better predictor of poor outcome when measured later during hospitalization compared with immediately after MI.

Measurement of NP plasma levels in combination with other biomarkers have potential benefits in the evaluation of risk and choice of therapeutic modality in acute coronary syndromes (ACSs; for selected references see Table 1). The data strongly suggest that CT-BNP and NT-BNP are independent indicators of mortality in ACSs for ACSs without ST-segment elevation and MI with ST-segment elevation [98,100–104]. Additionally, the determination of these markers could help to identify two subgroups of high-risk patients: those who do not have clinical signs of heart failure and those who do not have elevated levels of troponin [98,102]. In addition, the NPs are useful independent markers of mortality in the short and long term, independently of whether blood sampling is made upon admission or within hours or days of the onset of symptoms. In all cases, higher levels of BNP or NT-BNP were associated with increased mortality. This suggests that early determination would help in decision making in the acute phase [98,103,104]. The elevation of plasma NPs by themselves, or in association with other markers of risk, would be useful in deciding between an early invasive strategy or a noninvasive treatment, although some points need to be addressed (eg, influence of age, gender, assay systems, clinically relevant analyte range). In any event, troponin is best for the prognosis of recurrent ischemia and nonfatal MI. C-reactive protein or interleukin-6 detect active inflammation and the NPs are sensitive indicators of mortality. A combination of these markers could help in decision making. For example, patients with lower levels of troponin and NPs upon admission could benefit from a noninvasive strategy. Conversely, patients with high troponin, inflammation markers, and NPs would benefit from an early invasive strategy, because the markers denote a high risk for new ischemic events and increased mortality. There will patients with low levels of troponin and high levels of NPs. In these cases, the NPs would help to stratify them into the high-risk group, because high NP levels is a mortality marker that is independent of the course of the thrombotic event. The fundamental clinical question seems to be whether the NPs are elevated because they are a measure of mortality. Table 1 is a summary of some of the work concerning ACSs and NPs.

The studies that have compared measurements of NPs with other neuroendocrine variables, such as norepinephrine circulating levels, ANF, and BNP, showed the closest correlation to cardiovascular functional status [90,105]. It is tempting to speculate that in the early stages of heart failure, plasma renin activity and sympathetic activity are normal because the increased circulating levels of NPs suppress them. This might explain why NPs are elevated before other neuroendocrine variables are, and why the determination of NP plasma levels is an early and sensitive indicator of ventricular dysfunction.

The changes in NP secretion, as for example in studies that demonstrated an elevation of plasma NPs in subclinical systolic or diastolic dysfunction [87], are distinctive enough to make the measurements useful in diagnosis and prognosis beyond the group statistics (ie, they are useful adjuncts in the evaluation of the individual patient).

Acknowledgments

This work was supported by grants from the Canadian Institutes of Health Research and the Heart and Stroke Foundation of Ontario. The authors are grateful to Dr. Mercedes L Kuroski de Bold for providing the ultrastructural immunocytochemistry shown in Figure 2.

References

[1] de Bold AJ, Borenstein HB, Veress AT, et al. A rapid and potent natriuretic response to intravenous injection of atrial myocardial extracts in rats. Life Sci 1981;28:89–94.

[2] de Bold AJ. Atrial natriuretic factor: a hormone produced by the heart. Science 1985; 230:767–70.

[3] Maekawa K, Sudoh T, Furusawa M, et al. Cloning and sequence analysis of cDNA encoding a precursor for porcine brain natriuretic peptide. Biochem Biophys Res Commun 1988;157:410–6.

[4] Lincoln TM, Cornwell TL. Intracellular cyclic GMP receptor proteins. FASEB J 1993;7:328–38.

[5] Sano T, Morishita Y, Yamada K, et al. Effects of HS-142–1, a novel non-peptide ANP antagonist, on diuresis and natriuresis induced by acute volume expansion in anesthetized rats. Biochem Biophys Res Commun 1992;182:824–9.

[6] Sano T, Morishita Y, Matsuda Y, et al. Pharmacological profile of HS-142–1, a novel nonpeptide atrial natriuretic peptide antagonist of microbial

[7] Yokota N, Bruneau BG, Kuroski de Bold ML, et al. Atrial natriuretic factor significantly contributes to the mineralocorticoid escape phenomenon. Evidence for a guanylate cyclase-mediated pathway. J Clin Invest 1994;94:1938–46.

origin. I. Selective inhibition of the actions of natriuretic peptides in anesthetized rats. J Pharmacol Exp Ther 1992;260:825–31.

[8] John SW, Krege JH, Oliver PM, et al. Genetic decreases in atrial natriuretic peptide and salt-sensitive hypertension. Science 1995;267:679–81.

[9] Hill O, Kuhn M, Zucht HD, et al. Analysis of the human guanylin gene and the processing and cellular localization of the peptide. Proc Natl Acad Sci U S A 1995;92:2046–50.

[10] Oliver PM, Fox JE, Kim R, et al. Hypertension, cardiac hypertrophy, and sudden death in mice lacking natriuretic peptide receptor A. Proc Natl Acad Sci U S A 1997;94(26):14730–5.

[11] Ogawa Y, Tamura N, Chusho H, et al. Brain natriuretic peptide appears to act locally as an antifibrotic factor in the heart. Can J Physiol Pharmacol 2001;79:723–9.

[12] Christoffels VM, Keijser AG, Houweling AC, et al. Patterning the embryonic heart: identification of five mouse Iroquois homeobox genes in the developing heart. Dev Biol 2000;224:263–74.

[13] Houweling AC, Somi S, Massink MP, et al. Comparative analysis of the natriuretic peptide precursor gene cluster in vertebrates reveals loss of ANF and retention of CNP-3 in chicken. Dev Dyn 2005;233:1076–82.

[14] Kawakoshi A, Hyodo S, Inoue K, et al. Four natriuretic peptides (ANP, BNP, VNP and CNP) coexist in the sturgeon: identification of BNP in fish lineage. J Mol Endocrinol 2004;32:547–55.

[15] Sekiguchi T, Miyamoto K, Mizutani T, et al. Molecular cloning of natriuretic peptide receptor A from bullfrog (*Rana catesbeiana*) brain and its functional expression. Gene 2001;273:251–7.

[16] Argentin S, Sun Y, Lihrmann I, et al. Distal cis-acting promoter sequences mediate glucocorticoid stimulation of cardiac atrial natriuretic factor gene transcription. J Biol Chem 1991;266: 23315–22.

[17] Rockman HA, Ross RS, Harris AN, et al. Segregation of atrial-specific and inducible expression of an atrial natriuretic factor transgene in an in vivo murine model of cardiac hypertrophy. Proc Natl Acad Sci U S A 1991;88:8277–81.

[18] Engel JD, Beug H, LaVail JH, et al. Cis and trans regulation of tissue-specific transcription. J Cell Sci 1992;16:21–31.

[19] Sadoshima J, Jahn L, Takahashi T, et al. Molecular characterization of the stretch-induced adaptation of cultured cardiac cells. An in vitro model of load-induced cardiac hypertrophy. J Biol Chem 1992;267:10551–60.

[20] Kovacic-Milivojevic B, Gardner DG. Regulation of the human atrial natriuretic peptide gene in atrial cardiocytes by the transcription factor AP-1. Am J Hypertens 1993;6:258–63.

[21] Molkentin JD, Kalvakolanu DV, Markham BE. Transcription factor GATA-4 regulates cardiac muscle-specific expression of the alpha-myosin heavy-chain gene. Mol Cell Biol 1994;14:4947–57.

[22] Ogawa Y, Itoh H, Nakagawa O, et al. Characterization of the 5′-flanking region and chromosomal assignment of the human brain natriuretic peptide gene. J Mol Med 1995;73:457–63.

[23] Sprenkle AB, Murray SF, Glembotski CC. Involvement of multiple cis elements in basal- and alpha-adrenergic agonist-inducible atrial natriuretic factor transcription. Roles for serum response elements and an SP-1-like element. Circ Res 1995; 77:1060–9.

[24] Durocher D, Chen CY, Ardati A, et al. The atrial natriuretic factor promoter is a downstream target for Nkx-2.5 in the myocardium. Mol Cell Biol 1996;16:4648–55.

[25] LaPointe MC, Wu G, Garami M, et al. Tissue-specific expression of the human brain natriuretic peptide gene in cardiac myocytes. Hypertension 1996;27(Pt 2):715–22.

[26] Liang F, Gardner DG. Mechanical strain activates BNP gene transcription through a p38/NF-kappaB-dependent mechanism. J Clin Invest 1999;104:1603–12.

[27] Nicholas SB, Philipson KD. Cardiac expression of the Na$(^+)$/Ca(2^+) exchanger NCX1 is GATA factor dependent. Am J Physiol 1999;277:H324–30.

[28] Sarzani R, Dessi-Fulgheri P, Salvi F, et al. A novel promoter variant of the natriuretic peptide clearance receptor gene is associated with lower atrial natriuretic peptide and higher blood pressure in obese hypertensives. J Hypertens 1999;17: 1301–5.

[29] Liang F, Kovacic-Milivojevic B, Chen S, et al. Signaling mechanisms underlying strain-dependent brain natriuretic peptide gene transcription. Can J Physiol Pharmacol 2001;79:640–5.

[30] Marttila M, Hautala N, Paradis P, et al. GATA4 mediates activation of the B-type natriuretic peptide gene expression in response to hemodynamic stress. Endocrinology 2001;142:4693–700.

[31] McBride K, Nemer M. Regulation of the ANF and BNP promoters by GATA factors: lessons learned for cardiac transcription. Can J Physiol Pharmacol 2001;79:673–81.

[32] He Q, Mendez M, LaPointe MC. Regulation of the human brain natriuretic peptide gene by GATA-4. Am J Physiol Endocrinol Metab 2002;283:E50–7.

[33] Rubattu S, Giliberti R, De Paolis P, et al. Effect of a regulatory mutation on the rat atrial natriuretic peptide gene transcription. Peptides 2002;23: 555–60.

[34] Tomaru KK, Arai M, Yokoyama T, et al. Transcriptional activation of the BNP gene by lipopolysaccharide is mediated through GATA elements in neonatal rat cardiac myocytes. J Mol Cell Cardiol 2002;34:649–59.

[35] Anderson HD, Wang F, Gardner DG. Role of the epidermal growth factor receptor in signaling strain-dependent activation of the brain natriuretic peptide gene. J Biol Chem 2004;27:9287–97.

[36] Kim SH, Koh GY, Cho KW, et al. Stretch-activated atrial natriuretic peptide secretion in atria with heat shock protein 70 overexpression. Exp Biol Med (Maywood) 2003;228:200–6.

[37] Pikkarainen S, Tokola H, Kerkela R, et al. Endothelin-1-specific activation of B-type natriuretic peptide gene via p38 mitogen-activated protein kinase and nuclear ETS factors. J Biol Chem 2003;278:3969–75.

[38] Kathiriya IS, King IN, Murakami M, et al. Hairy-related transcription factors inhibit GATA-dependent cardiac gene expression through a signal-responsive mechanism. J Biol Chem 2004; 279:54937–43.

[39] Ma KK, Ogawa T, de Bold AJ. Selective upregulation of cardiac brain natriuretic peptide at the transcriptional and translational levels by pro-inflammatory cytokines and by conditioned medium derived from mixed lymphocyte reactions via p38 MAP kinase. J Mol Cell Cardiol 2004;36: 505–13.

[40] Small EM, Krieg PA. Molecular regulation of cardiac chamber-specific gene expression. Trends Cardiovasc Med 2004;14:13–8.

[41] Toro R, Saadi I, Kuburas A, et al. Cell-specific activation of the atrial natriuretic factor promoter by PITX2 and MEF2A. J Biol Chem 2004;279: 52087–94.

[42] LaPointe MC. Molecular regulation of the brain natriuretic peptide gene. Peptides 2005;26:944–56.

[43] Ma KK, Banas K, de Bold AJ. Determinants of inducible brain natriuretic peptide promoter activity. Regul Pept 2005;128(3):169–76.

[44] Bloch KD, Seidman JG, Naftilan JD, et al. Neonatal atria and ventricles secrete atrial natriuretic factor via tissue-specific secretory pathways. Cell 1986;47:695–702.

[45] Zeller R, Bloch KD, Williams BS, et al. Localized expression of the atrial natriuretic factor gene during cardiac embryogenesis. Genes Dev 1987;1: 693–8.

[46] Lee RT, Bloch KD, Pfeffer JM, et al. Atrial natriuretic factor gene expression in ventricles of rats with spontaneous biventricular hypertrophy. J Clin Invest 1988;81:431–4.

[47] Rosenzweig A, Halazonetis TD, Seidman JG, et al. Proto-oncogenes c-fos/c-jun bind a Cis-control element of the atrial natriuretic factor gene [abstract]. J Clin Endocrinol Metab 1990;1:1.

[48] Seidman CE, Schmidt EV, Seidman JG. cis-dominance of rat atrial natriuretic factor gene regulatory sequences in transgenic mice. Can J Physiol Pharmacol 1991;69:1486–92.

[49] Bruneau BG, Nemer G, Schmitt JP, et al. A murine model of Holt-Oram syndrome defines roles of the T-box transcription factor Tbx5 in cardiogenesis and disease. Cell 2001;106:709–21.

[50] Bruneau BG, Bao ZZ, Fatkin D, et al. Cardiomyopathy in Irx4-deficient mice is preceded by abnormal ventricular gene expression. Mol Cell Biol 2001;21:1730–6.

[51] Ruskoaho H. Cardiac hormones as diagnostic tools in heart failure. Endocr Rev 2003;24:341–56.

[52] Sudoh T, Maekawa K, Kojima M, et al. Cloning and sequence analysis of cDNA encoding a precursor for human brain natriuretic peptide. Biochem Biophys Res Commun 1989;159:1427–34.

[53] Yokota N, Bruneau BG, Fernandez BE, et al. Dissociation of cardiac hypertrophy, myosin heavy chain isoform expression, and natriuretic peptide production in DOCA-salt rats. Am J Hypertens 1995;8:301–10.

[54] Ogawa T, Vatta M, Bruneau BG, et al. Characterization of natriuretic peptide production by adult heart atria. Am J Physiol Heart Circ Physiol 1999;276:H1977–86.

[55] Yao J, Suwa M, Li B, et al. ATP-dependent mechanism for coordination of intercellular Ca^{2+} signaling and renin secretion in rat juxtaglomerular cells. Circ Res 2003;93:338–45.

[56] Yatsu T, Kurosawa H, Hayashi M, et al. The role of $Ca2^{+}$ in the control of renin release from dog renal cortical slices. Eur J Pharmacol 2003;458:191–6.

[57] de Bold AJ, de Bold ML. Factors affecting cardionatrin release. In: Christiansen C, Riis BJ, editors. Highlights in endocrinology. Copenhagen (Denmark): N. Bogtrykkeri; 1987. p. 161–3.

[58] Katoh S, Toyama J, Aoyama M, et al. Mechanisms of atrial natriuretic peptide (ANP) secretion by rat hearts perfused in vitro–$Ca2^{+}$-dependent signal transduction for ANP release by mechanical stretch. Jap Circ J 1990;54:1283–94.

[59] Cho KW, Seul KH, Kim SH, et al. Atrial pressure, distension, and pacing frequency in ANP secretion in isolated perfused rabbit atria. Am J Physiol 1991; 260:R39–46.

[60] Kuroski de Bold ML, de Bold AJ. Stretch-secretion coupling in atrial cardiocytes. Dissociation between atrial natriuretic factor release and mechanical activity. Hypertension 1991;18:III-169–78.

[61] Mangat H, de Bold AJ. Stretch-induced atrial natriuretic factor release utilizes a rapidly depleting pool of newly synthesized hormone. Endocrinology 1993;133:1398–403.

[62] Arvan P, Castle JD. Phasic release of newly synthesized secretory proteins in the unstimulated rat exocrine pancreas. J Cell Biol 1987;104:243–52.

[63] Arvan P, Kuliawat R, Prabakaran D, et al. Protein discharge from immature secretory granules displays both regulated and constitutive characteristics. J Biol Chem 1991;266:14171–4.

[64] Kuliawat R, Arvan P. Protein targeting via the "constitutive-like" secretory pathway in isolated pancreatic islets: passive sorting in the immature granule compartment. J Cell Biol 1992;118: 521–9.

[65] Bensimon M, Chang A, Kuroski-de Bold ML, et al. Participation of G proteins in natriuretic peptide hormone secretion from heart atria. Endocrinology 2004;145:5313–21.

[66] de Bold AJ, Ma KK, Zhang Y, et al. The physiological and pathophysiological modulation of the endocrine function of the heart. Can J Physiol Pharmacol 2001;79:705–14.

[67] Miki K, Hajduczok G, Klocke MR, et al. Atrial natriuretic factor and renal function during head-out water immersion in conscious dogs. Am J Physiol 1986;251(5 Pt 2):R1000–4.

[68] Miki K, Shiraki K, Sagawa S, et al. Atrial natriuretic factor during head-out immersion at night. Am J Physiol 1988;254:R235–41.

[69] de Bold AJ, Bruneau BG, de Bold ML. Mechanical and neuroendocrine regulation of the endocrine heart. Cardiovasc Res 1996;31:7–18.

[70] Koller PT, Grekin RJ, Nicklas JM. Paradoxical response of plasma atrial natriuretic hormone to pericardiocentesis in cardiac tamponade. Am J Cardiol 1987;59:491–2.

[71] Northridge DB, McMurray J, Ray S, et al. Release of atrial natriuretic factor after pericardiocentesis for malignant pericardial effusion. BMJ 1989;299: 603–4.

[72] Uusimaa PA, Hassinen IE, Vuolteenaho O, et al. Endothelin-induced atrial natriuretic peptide release from cultured neonatal cardiac myocytes: the role of extracellular calcium and protein kinase-C. Endocrinology 1992;130:2455–64.

[73] Li Q, Gardner DG. Negative regulation of the human atrial natriuretic peptide gene by 1,25-dihydroxyvitamin D3. J Biol Chem 1994;269: 4934–9.

[74] Bianciotti LG, Vatta MS, Vescina C, et al. Centrally applied atrial natriuretic factor diminishes bile secretion in the rat. Regul Pept 2001;102: 127–33.

[75] Bianciotti LG, de Bold AJ. Natriuretic peptide gene expression in DOCA-salt hypertension after blockade of type B endothelin receptor. Am J Physiol Heart Circ Physiol 2002;282:H1127–34.

[76] Ogawa T, Linz W, Stevenson M, et al. Evidence for load-dependent and load-independent determinants of cardiac natriuretic peptide production. Circulation 1996;93:2059–67.

[77] Bianciotti LG, de Bold AJ. Modulation of cardiac natriuretic peptide gene expression following endothelin type A receptor blockade in renovascular hypertension. Cardiovasc Res 2001;49:808–16.

[78] Masters RG, Davies RA, Keon WJ, et al. Neuroendocrine response to cardiac transplantation. Can J Cardiol 1993;9:609–17.

[79] Masters RG, Davies RA, Veinot JP, et al. Discoordinate modulation of natriuretic peptides during acute cardiac allograft rejection in humans. Circulation 1999;100:287–91.

[80] Ogawa T, Veinot JP, Davies RA, et al. Neuroendocrine profiling of humans receiving cardiac allografts. J Heart Lung Transplant 2005;24:1046–54.

[81] Murakami Y, Shimada T, Inoue S, et al. New insights into the mechanism of the elevation of plasma brain natriuretic polypeptide levels in patients with left ventricular hypertrophy. Can J Cardiol 2002;18:1294–300.

[82] Cody RJ, Atlas SA, Laragh JH, et al. Atrial natriuretic factor in normal subjects and heart failure patients. Plasma levels and renal, hormonal, and hemodynamic responses to peptide infusion. J Clin Invest 1986;78:1362–74.

[83] Chen HH, Burnett JC. Natriuretic peptides in the pathophysiology of congestive heart failure. Curr Cardiol Rep 2000;2:198–205.

[84] Hall C, Cannon CP, Forman S, et al. Prognostic value of N-terminal proatrial natriuretic factor plasma levels measured within the first 12 hours after myocardial infarction. J Am Coll Cardiol 1995; 26(6):1452–6.

[85] Motwani JG, McAlpine H, Kennedy N, et al. Plasma brain natriuretic peptide as an indicator for angiotensin-converting enzyme inhibition after myocardial infarction. Lancet 1993;341:1109–13.

[86] Lerman A, Gibbons RJ, Rodeheffer RJ, et al. Circulating N-terminal atrial natriuretic peptide as a marker for symptomless left-ventricular dysfunction. Lancet 1993;341:1105–9.

[87] Arad M, Elazar E, Shotan A, et al. Brain and atrial natriuretic peptides in patients with ischemic heart disease with and without heart failure. Cardiology 1996;87:12–7.

[88] Richards AM, Crozier IG, Yandle TG, et al. Brain natriuretic factor: regional plasma concentrations and correlations with haemodynamic state in cardiac disease. Br Heart J 1993;69:414–7.

[89] Davis KM, Fish LC, Elahi D, et al. Atrial natriuretic peptide levels in the prediction of congestive heart failure risk in frail elderly. JAMA 1992;267: 2625–9.

[90] Dickstein K, Larsen AI, Bonarjee V, et al. Plasma proatrial natriuretic factor is predictive of clinical status in patients with congestive heart failure. Am J Cardiol 1995;76:679–83.

[91] Moe GW, Rouleau JL, Charbonneau L, et al. Neurohormonal activation in severe heart failure: relations to patient death and the effect of treatment with flosequinan. Am Heart J 2000;139(4): 587–95.

[92] Bastos R, Favaretto AL, Gutkowska J, et al. Alpha-adrenergic agonists inhibit the dipsogenic effect of angiotensin II by their stimulation of atrial natriuretic peptide release. Brain Res 2001;895: 80–8.

[93] Maisel AS. Practical approaches to treating patients with acute decompensated heart failure. J Card Fail 2001;7:13–7.

[94] Dao Q, Krishnaswamy P, Kazanegra R, et al. Utility of B-type natriuretic peptide in the diagnosis of congestive heart failure in an urgent-care setting. J Am Coll Cardiol 2001;37:379–85.

[95] Kazanegra R, Cheng V, Garcia A, et al. A rapid test for B-type natriuretic peptide correlates with falling wedge pressures in patients treated for decompensated heart failure: a pilot study. J Card Fail 2001;7:21–9.

[96] Maisel A. B-type natriuretic peptide levels: a potential novel "white count" for congestive heart failure. J Card Fail 2001;7:183–93.

[97] Cheng V, Kazanagra R, Garcia A, et al. A rapid bedside test for B-type peptide predicts treatment outcomes in patients admitted for decompensated heart failure: a pilot study. J Am Coll Cardiol 2001;37:386–91.

[98] de Lemos JA, Morrow DA, Bentley JH, et al. The prognostic value of B-type natriuretic peptide in patients with acute coronary syndromes. N Engl J Med 2001;345:1014–21.

[99] Talwar S, Squire IB, Downie PF, et al. Profile of plasma N-terminal proBNP following acute myocardial infarction. Eur Heart J 2000;21: 1514–21.

[100] James SK, Lindahl B, Siegbahn A, et al. N-terminal pro-brain natriuretic peptide and other risk markers for the separate prediction of mortality and subsequent myocardial infarction in patients with unstable coronary artery disease: a Global Utilization of Strategies To Open occluded arteries (GUSTO)-IV substudy. Circulation 2003;108: 275–81.

[101] Morrow DA, de Lemos JA, Sabatine MS, et al. Evaluation of B-type natriuretic peptide for risk assessment in unstable angina/non-ST-elevation myocardial infarction: B-type natriuretic peptide and prognosis in TACTICS-TIMI 18. J Am Coll Cardiol 2003;41:1264–72.

[102] Omland T, Persson A, Ng L, et al. N-terminal pro-B-type natriuretic peptide and long-term mortality in acute coronary syndromes. Circulation 2002; 106:2913–8.

[103] Jernberg T, Stridsberg M, Lindahl B. Usefulness of plasma N-terminal proatrial natriuretic peptide (proANP) as an early predictor of outcome in unstable angina pectoris or non-ST-elevation acute myocardial infarction. Am J Cardiol 2002;89: 64–6.

[104] Galvani M, Ferrini D, Ottani F. Natriuretic peptides for risk stratification of patients with acute coronary syndromes. Eur J Heart Fail 2004;6: 327–33.

[105] Hall C, Rouleau JL, Moyé L, et al. N-terminal proatrial natriuretic factor. Circulation 1994;89: 1934–42.

[106] Flynn TG, de Bold AJ, de Bold ML, et al. Main forms of immunoreactive cardionatrin in atrial extracts and in atrial specific granules. Biochem Soc Trans 1985;13:1141.

[107] Casco VH, Veinot JP, Kuroski de Bold ML, et al. Natriuretic peptide system gene expression in human coronary arteries. J Histochem Cytochem 2002;50:799–809.

[108] Fontana F, Bernardi P, Spagnolo N, et al. Plasma atrial natriuretic factor in patients with acute myocardial infarction. Eur Heart J 1990;11: 779–87.

[109] Ngo L, Vesely DL, Bissett JK, et al. Acute and sustained release of the atrial natriuretic factor prohormone N-terminus with acute myocardial infarction. Am J Med Sci 1991;301:157–64.

[110] Morita E, Yasue H, Yoshimura M, et al. Increased plasma levels of brain natriuretic peptide in patients with acute myocardial infarction. Circulation 1993; 88:82–91.

[111] Horio T, Shimada K, Kohno M, et al. Serial changes in atrial and brain natriuretic peptides in patients with acute myocardial infarction treated with early coronary angioplasty. Am Heart J 1993;126:293–9.

[112] Omland T, de Lemos JA, Morrow DA, et al. Prognostic value of N-terminal pro-atrial and pro-brain natriuretic peptide in patients with acute coronary syndromes. Am J Cardiol 2002;89:463–5.

[113] Jernberg T, Lindahl B, Siegbahn A, et al. N-terminal pro-brain natriuretic peptide in relation to inflammation, myocardial necrosis, and the effect of an invasive strategy in unstable coronary artery disease. J Am Coll Cardiol 2003;42: 1909–16.

[114] Galvani M, Ottani F, Oltrona L, et al. N-terminal pro-brain natriuretic peptide on admission has prognostic value across the whole spectrum of acute coronary syndromes. Circulation 2004;110: 128–34.

[115] Heeschen C, Hamm CW, Mitrovic V, et al. N-terminal pro-B-type natriuretic peptide levels for dynamic risk stratification of patients with acute coronary syndromes. Circulation 2004;110: 3206–12.

[116] Lindahl B, Lindback J, Jernberg T, et al. Serial analyses of N-terminal pro-B-type natriuretic peptide in patients with non-ST-segment elevation acute coronary syndromes: a Fragmin and fast Revascularisation during In Stability in Coronary artery disease (FRISC)-II substudy. J Am Coll Cardiol 2005;45:533–41.

[117] Morrow DA, de Lemos JA, Blazing MA, et al. Prognostic value of serial B-type natriuretic

peptide testing during follow-up of patients with unstable coronary artery disease. JAMA 2005; 294:2866–71.

[118] Bjorklund E, Jernberg T, Johanson P, et al. Admission N-terminal pro-brain natriuretic peptide and its interaction with admission troponin T and ST segment resolution for early risk stratification in ST elevation myocardial infarction. Heart 2006; 92:735–40.

[119] James SK, Lindahl B, Timmer JR, et al. Usefulness of biomarkers for predicting long-term mortality in patients with diabetes mellitus and non-ST-elevation acute coronary syndromes (a GUSTO IV substudy). Am J Cardiol 2006;97:167–72.

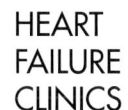

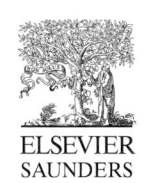

Natriuretic Peptides as Regulators of Myocardial Structure and Function: Pathophysiologic and Therapeutic Implications

Alessandro Cataliotti, MD, PhD*, Horng H. Chen, MBBCh, Margaret M. Redfield, MD, John C. Burnett, Jr, MD

Mayo Clinic, Rochester, MN, USA

The longstanding conventional view of the natriuretic peptide system is one in which the natriuretic peptides form an important cardiorenal endocrine axis. Specifically, the heart synthesizes and releases atrial natriuretic peptide (ANP) and brain natriuretic peptide (BNP) that function to optimize intravascular volume and arterial pressure. This homeostatic function is mediated by renal, vascular, and endocrine actions that adapt to the volume status of the individual. This article diverges from this concept and advances an emerging paradigm for the natriuretic peptides as a regulator of cardiac structure and function [1]. Most importantly, the authors review new knowledge that underscores that the natriuretic peptide system functions to maintain myocardial structure and function through actions on cardiomyocytes and nonmyocytes. Such cardiac properties are important in cardiac development as well as having therapeutic relevance in cardiovascular disease. Indeed, as discussed herein, evidence is emerging in heart failure and hypertension that there may be a deficiency of biologically active natriuretic peptides, arguing for the use of the natriuretic peptides as therapy to maintain optimal myocardial structure and function.

This work was supported by grants from the National Institutes of Health (PO1HL76611, HL36634, and HL83231) and the Mayo Foundation.
* Corresponding author. Cardiorenal Research Laboratory, Division of Cardiovascular Diseases, Mayo Clinic, 200 First Street SW, Rochester, MN 55904.
 E-mail address: cataliotti.alessandro@mayo.edu (A. Cataliotti).

Natriuretic peptides and cardiomyocyte function

The importance of the natriuretic peptides in the control of myocardial structure is strongly suggested by studies of cardiac development. Peaks of expression of ANP and BNP occur with significant events in cardiac organogenesis, supporting a role for these cardiac hormones in the formation of the heart [2]. Indeed, in mice lacking the natriuretic peptide receptor A (NPRA) gene (Npr1$^{-/-}$), survival is reduced with hearts enlarged at birth and possible cardiac developmental abnormalities [3,4]. The adult phenotype of such mice is elevated blood pressure and marked cardiac hypertrophy and fibrosis, indicating that the natriuretic peptide system has an important role in cardiomyocyte growth and development.

The increase in myocardial load that occurs with hypertension in NPRA or ANP gene disruptions makes interpretation of the findings in such genetically altered mice difficult from the perspective of understanding the direct actions of the natriuretic peptides on cardiomyocyte growth and function. Furthermore, the low density of NPRA in cardiomyocytes has raised the question of the importance of these receptors in the modulation of cardiomyocytes when compared with the markedly higher expression levels that are observed in the kidneys and adrenals. Despite a relative low concentration of NPRA in the heart as compared with other tissues, mounting evidence underscores the important role of this receptor in regulating the antigrowth and antifibrotic actions of the cardiac peptides ANP and

BNP. In elegant studies by Holtwick and coworkers [5], mice with cardiac specific disruption of the NPRA demonstrated impaired relaxation and exaggerated hypertrophic responses to pressure overload, supporting a key role for the natriuretic peptide system as a regulator of myocardial structure and function. Indeed, the impaired relaxation during NPRA cardiac specific disruption is consistent with observations that, when infused in a large animal model of heart failure, both ANP and BNP result in enhanced ventricular relaxation with an improvement in diastolic function [6].

The authors have taken advantage of continuing insights into the biology of the NPRA. Specifically, the NPRA receptor is composed of extracellular ligand binding, transmembrane, protein kinase–like, hinge, and catalytic domains [7]. It is well established that receptor homodimerization and ATP binding are required for guanylyl cyclase activity. Furthermore, the region required for homodimer formation resides in the carboxy terminal portion of the HCAT (hinge and catalytic domain). A dominant negative form of the NPRA receptor (DN-NPRA) could be a result of the recruitment of homodimer formation. Specifically, a truncated form of NPRA containing only the HCAT domain heterodimerizes with wild-type NPRA, resulting in attenuated NPRA activity and cGMP generation to ANP.

The authors developed mice cardiac specific expression of the DN-NPRA to further investigate the autocrine and paracrine actions of the natriuretic peptide system in the heart [8]. The specific hypothesis was that DN-NPRA mice would demonstrate alterations in cardiac structure and function in the absence of alterations in blood pressure when exposed to pressure overload produced by aortic banding. In the absence of pressure overload, basal and BNP stimulated guanylyl cyclase activity was reduced; however, blood pressure, myocardial cGMP, ANP, and myocardial structure and function were normal in the DN-NPRA mice when compared with wild-type mice. In the presence of pressure overload, myocardial cGMP was reduced, and ventricular filling pressures were increased in association with greater ventricular hypertrophy, fibrosis, and mortality in the DN-NPRA mice when compared with wild-types. These studies, which are similar to the work of Holtwick and colleagues, support the conclusion that the endogenous natriuretic peptide system exerts physiologically relevant autocrine and paracrine effects via cardiomyocyte NPRA receptors to modulate cardiac hypertrophy and fibrosis in response to pressure overload.

The molecular mechanism of natriuretic peptide regulation of cardiomyocyte growth is only now emerging. To address this issue, Tokudome and coworkers [9] investigated the role of calcineurin, a calcium-dependent phosphatase, in cardiac remodeling in NPRA knockout (KO) mice. They first observed that in the hearts of young NPRA KO mice, calcineurin activity, nuclear translocation of nuclear factor of activated T cells c3 (NFATc3), and modulatory calcineurin-interacting protein 1 (MCIP1) gene expressions were increased when compared with wild-type mice. Inhibition of calcineurin activity by FK506 decreased the heart to body weight ratio, cardiomyocyte size, and collagen volume fraction, whereas such inhibition had no impact in wild-type mice. The findings supported the concept that activation of NPRA by locally secreted natriuretic peptides protects the heart from excessive cardiomyocyte hypertrophy by inhibition of the calcineurin-NFATc3 pathway. Complementing a role of the calcineurin-NFATc3 pathway in the regulation of cardiomyocyte growth by the natriuretic peptides is the report by Silberbach and coworkers [10] suggesting that there is also an important linkage between cGMP signaling and the mitogen-activated protein kinase cascade, and that selective ANP activation of ERK is required for the antihypertrophic action of this natriuretic peptide.

Kato and colleagues [11] have recently advanced the understanding of yet another paracrine/autocrine role of the natriuretic peptides, that is, the property of mediating cardiomyocyte survival. Specifically, they reported that ANP at a dose of 10^{-9} M mediated anti-apoptotic signaling via cGMP and subsequent nuclear accumulation of Akt kinase associated with zyxin, a cytoskeletal LIM-domain protein in vitro. Nuclear targeting of zyxin induced resistance to cell death in association with nuclear accumulation of activated Akt. Potentiation of cell survival was induced by ANP or cGMP signaling. Myocardial nuclear accumulation of zyxin and Akt responded similarly in vivo following treatment of mice with ANP or cGMP. It was concluded that zyxin and activated Akt participate in a cGMP-dependent signaling cascade following ANP stimulation of NPRA receptors to nuclear accumulation of both molecules. Nuclear accumulation of zyxin and activated Akt may represent a fundamental mechanism that facilitates nuclear signal transduction and potentiates cell survival.

Natriuretic peptides and cardiac fibroblasts

The cardiac interstitium is a dynamic structure as reflected by continuous synthesis and degradation of matrix proteins. The family of matrix metalloproteinases (MMPs) consists of more than 20 different zinc-containing, Ca^{2+}-dependent endopeptidases that degrade matrix proteins and has an important role in the physiologic regulation of the interstitium. It is now well recognized that cardiac fibroblasts have a critical regulatory role in control of the cardiac extracellular matrix by synthesizing collagen and other matrix proteins as well as by promoting their degradation by secreting MMP proteins. Cameron and coworkers [12] recently reported that ANP is produced in cardiac fibroblasts after myocardial infarction, indicating that fibroblasts, like cardiomyocytes, can be a source of natriuretic peptides. Until recently, it remained unknown whether BNP was produced by cardiac fibroblasts.

The authors recently investigated whether cardiac fibroblasts produce BNP and whether BNP and its signaling system contribute to the regulation of collagen synthesis and the activation of MMPs [13]. In these studies, BNP mRNA was detected in cardiac fibroblasts, and a specific radioimmunoassay demonstrated that BNP1-32 was secreted from these cells. The amount of BNP secretion was significantly augmented by tumor necrosis factor. BNP inhibited de novo collagen synthesis, whereas zymographic MMP-2 (gelatinase) abundance was stimulated by BNP. In addition, protein expression of MMP-1, -2, and -3 and membranous type-1 MMP was increased by BNP. The cGMP analogue 8-bromo-cGMP mimicked the BNP effect, whereas inhibition of protein kinase G by KT5823 attenuated BNP-induced zymographic MMP-2 abundance. These in vitro findings support a role for BNP as a regulator of myocardial structure via control of cardiac fibroblast function. More recently, Calderone and coworkers [14] extended our studies to localize ANP and BNP in cardiac fibroblasts associated with scar formation following acute myocardial infarction. They observed that ANP and BNP mRNA levels were significantly increased in the noninfarcted left ventricle and scar of 1-week post myocardial infarction male rats when compared with the levels in the left ventricle of normal rats. Following 4 to 7 days in culture, myofibroblasts expressed organized alpha-smooth muscle actin filaments; however, natriuretic peptides were predominantly detected in the nucleus and cytoplasm, and thin filaments occupying the perinuclear region were positive for preproANP and BNP. It was concluded that natriuretic peptide synthesis by cardiac myofibroblasts may in part influence reparative fibrosis.

Evidence supporting a functionally important antifibrotic property of the natriuretic peptides is their interaction with the profibrotic cytokine transforming growth factor-beta (TGF-beta). Kapoun and coworkers [15] reported that BNP inhibited TGF-beta-induced cell proliferation as well as the production of collagen 1 and fibronectin proteins as measured by Western blot analysis. Elegant cDNA microarray analysis was performed on cardiac fibroblasts incubated in the presence or absence of TGF-beta and BNP. BNP treatment reduced the effects of TGF-beta. Specifically, 88% and 85% of all TGF-beta-regulated mRNAs were affected at 24 and 48 hours, respectively. Furthermore, BNP inhibited TGF-beta–regulated genes related to fibrosis (collagen 1, fibronectin, CTGF, PAI-1, and TIMP3), myofibroblast conversion (alpha-smooth muscle actin 2 and nonmuscle myosin heavy chain), proliferation (PDGFA, IGF1, FGF18, and IGFBP10), and inflammation (COX2, IL6, TNF-alpha–induced protein 6, and TNF superfamily member 4). These studies strongly support the conclusion that BNP has a direct effect on cardiac fibroblasts to inhibit fibrotic responses, suggesting that BNP functions as an antifibrotic factor in the heart to prevent cardiac remodeling in pathologic conditions.

As discussed previously, cardiac remodeling involves the accumulation of extracellular matrix proteins including fibronectin. It has been recognized that fibronectin contains RGD motifs that bind integrins at DDX sequences, allowing signaling from the extracellular matrix to the nucleus. The authors noted that the NPRA sequence also contains RGD and DDX sequences; therefore, studies were performed to determine whether there could be cross talk between the extracellular matrix and BNP in cardiac fibroblasts by investigating potential interactions between fibronectin and NPRA on BNP induction of cGMP in cardiac fibroblasts. A further goal was to determine whether this interaction could be augmented with a Mayo designed NPRA specific RGD peptide that could then have therapeutic potential in the prevention of cardiac fibrosis as a small molecule [16]. Cardiac fibroblasts placed on fibronectin-coated plates demonstrated a pronounced increase in cGMP production to BNP when compared with noncoated plates. This cGMP production was also enhanced by the NPRA specific RGD peptide. Furthermore, a possible role was defined for the NPRC receptor through a non-cGMP mechanism in mediating the antiproliferative actions of BNP in cardiac fibroblasts wherein the NPRC receptor antagonist blocked BNP inhibition of proliferation in these cells. The evidence is strong that BNP and most likely ANP and the C-type natriuretic peptide are potent antifibrotic peptides with therapeutic potential in the inhibition of cardiac fibrosis, warranting further studies.

Although the studies discussed previously are largely in vitro investigations, one seminal in vivo study strongly supports the interaction between the natriuretic peptides and modulation of the extracellular matrix of the heart. Tamura and coworkers [17] developed mice with targeted disruption of BNP. They observed multifocal fibrotic lesions in the ventricles from BNP KO mice. Interestingly, unlike in the ANP KO mice, no systemic hypertension or ventricular hypertrophy was noted; however, in response to ventricular pressure overload, focal fibrotic lesions were markedly increased to a greater extent than observed in wild-type mice. When this study is taken together with studies in cultured cardiac fibroblasts, one may conclude that BNP is an antifibrotic factor in vivo, providing evidence for its role as a local regulator of ventricular structure and function independently of cardiac load and pressure.

Deficiencies of natriuretic peptides in cardiovascular disease

The conventional view of circulating natriuretic peptides in cardiovascular disease is that they are elevated and serve as exceptional biomarkers, especially in heart failure. This view is beginning to evolve as mounting evidence suggests that BNP circulates in different structural forms. Recently, the authors developed and used an immunoaffinity purification assay to isolate endogenous BNP1-32 from the plasma of New York Heart Association class IV patients for subsequent analysis by nano-liquid chromatography (LC) electrospray ionization Fourier transform ion cyclotron resonance (FT-ICR) MS [18]. Stable isotope-labeled BNP1-32 was introduced to the assayed plasma to enable quantification of endogenous levels of BNP1-32. Unlike the chemically nonspecific point-of-care tests (POCTs) and radioimmunoassays used worldwide to quantify BNP1-32 from plasma, FT-ICR-MS (with unprecedented mass measurement accuracy) coupled with LC (retention time) affords extraordinary molecular specificity. When combined with the use of internal standards, it can confidently identify and quantify BNP1-32. Despite exceedingly high circulating levels of BNP1-32 in the New York Heart Association class IV patients as determined by POCTs, nano-LC-electrospray ionization-FT-ICR-MS data did not reveal any endogenous BNP1-32. These results provide molecularly specific evidence for the absence of circulating BNP1-32 in advanced stage heart failure patients and suggest the existence of altered forms of BNP that are contributing to the POCT values.

Although other immunoreactive BNP forms in advanced heart failure may replace BNP1-32, evidence suggests a lack of or genetically altered activation of the natriuretic peptide system in human hypertension contributing to a relative deficiency. Such a deficiency could have major implications and contribute to adverse cardiac remodeling as well as further elevation of arterial pressure owing to the lack of cardiovascular protection provided by the endogenous natriuretic peptides. Recently, Belluardo and coworkers [19] evaluated the relationship between two circulating molecular forms of BNP (BNP1-32 and NT-proBNP), the severity of hypertension, and cardiac hypertrophy in subjects with mild, moderate, and severe hypertension. In grade 1 hypertension, BNP1-32 was not elevated and NT-proBNP was reduced when compared with controls, suggesting that early stages of hypertension are characterized by a lack of activation of the cardiac protective system of BNP.

Elegant work by Dries and coworkers [20] has revealed the existence of a corin gene allele defined by two missense mutations that is associated with hypertension. Corin cleaves ANP and BNP into smaller biologically active molecules, and its genetic alteration or maladaptive modulation by hypertension could suppress the activation and processing of ANP and BNP with pathophysiologic consequences. This effect has been clearly shown in corin-deficient (Cor$^{-/-}$) mice. Cor$^{-/-}$ mice have elevated levels of proANP but no detectable levels of mature ANP [21]. Using radiotelemetry to assess blood pressure, Cor$^{-/-}$ mice had spontaneous hypertension when compared with wild-type mice, which was enhanced after dietary salt loading. These data and the findings of

Dries establish corin as the physiologic pronatriuretic peptide convertase and indicate that a corin deficiency may contribute to hypertensive heart disease.

A compelling study linking the natriuretic peptides and cardiac structure has been reported by Rubattu and coworkers [22]. These investigators addressed the relationship between the natriuretic peptides and cardiac mass in human hypertension, exploring the possibility of an ANP deficiency based on ANP polymorphisms. They specifically focused on hypertensive subjects carrying the ANP gene promoter allelic variant and found that they demonstrated an increased left ventricular mass index and relative wall thickening when compared with the wild-type genotype. These carriers also demonstrated significantly lower plasma proANP levels when compared with heterozygote subjects. These studies strongly support the existence of genetic derangements in human hypertension for the natriuretic peptide system that may have important functional relevance to the development and treatment of cardiac hypertrophy and fibrosis.

Therapeutic implications for natriuretic peptide therapy to preserve myocardial structure and function: novel indications, delivery strategies, and innovative new generation peptides

Acute myocardial infarction

Acute myocardial infarction is a complication of coronary artery disease and may lead to loss of ventricular myocardium with cardiac enlargement and fibrosis because the heart cannot regenerate itself. Strong evidence suggests that the cardiac natriuretic peptides ANP and BNP are small endogenous hormones possessing cardioprotective properties that may protect the heart from injury, preserving cardiac structure and function. Evidence is emerging to support the therapeutic application of ANP and BNP in human acute myocardial infarction as an approach in cardioprotection [23]. Complementing the direct actions on the cardiomyocyte and cardiac fibroblast by ANP and BNP via cGMP are their ability to mediate coronary vasodilatation and reduce myocardial oxygen consumption, enhance myocardial relaxation, suppress aldosterone release, including aldosterone synthesis in cultured cardiomyocytes, retard adrenergic activation, and induce vascular regeneration [6,24–28]. Based in part on the elegant human studies of Hayashi and coworkers [29], two human clinical trials are ongoing in the United States and Japan to test the hypothesis that BNP and ANP, respectively, infused at the time of acute myocardial infarction without heart failure for 3 days can preserve myocardial structure and function and reduce the ultimate development of human heart failure.

Oral brain natriuretic peptide

Oral administration of intact and biologically active peptides has long been a therapeutic challenge. Most recently, new technologies have been developed that may be instrumental in achieving this objective. The authors and others recently applied these new technologies to BNP. First, in experimental hypertension, administration of long-acting BNP synthesized as a fusion peptide with albumin resulted in sustained blood pressure–lowering actions, supporting a strategy for longer-term BNP therapy in cardiovascular diseases, especially hypertension, in which BNP or ANP may be deficient, and the cardiac phenotype is hypertrophy and fibrosis with diastolic dysfunction [30].

To move toward oral BNP, the authors have employed proprietary technology (Nobex) in which short amphiphilic oligomers are covalently attached to peptides. In contrast to standard PEGylation technology, this technique employs comparatively small amphiphilic oligomers that are monodispersed and comprise both a hydrophobic (alkyl) moiety and a hydrophilic polyethylene glycol (PEG) moiety. The oligomers are intended to improve the pharmacokinetic and pharmacodynamic profiles of the peptide and enable oral administration.

The authors addressed the feasibility and the biologic activity of acute orally administered conjugated BNP (CONJ-BNP) [31]. These studies evaluated for the first time a novel form of CONJ-hBNP (hBNP-021) through oral administration. In a randomized crossover-designed study, the biologic activity of oral CONJ-BNP was tested and compared with that of oral native BNP in normal conscious dogs. Measurements of mean arterial pressure (MAP), plasma BNP, and cGMP were made at baseline and repeated at 10, 30, 60, 120, 180, and 240 minutes after oral administration. As expected, plasma human BNP was not detectable in dogs at baseline, whereas plasma human BNP that was used for oral BNP was detected after CONJ-hBNP administration. Importantly, plasma human BNP concentration was significantly higher after CONJ-BNP administration. Plasma cGMP increased after CONJ-hBNP for 60 minutes, whereas it did not change after native hBNP. MAP decreased at 10 minutes and remained decreased for 60 minutes after CONJ-hBNP while remaining unchanged after native hBNP. This study clearly demonstrated that BNP is absorbed intact and promotes sustained biologic actions when administered orally as a conjugated form. These data suggest the importance of pursuing further studies with oral administration of conjugated forms of human BNP for the long-term treatment of cardiovascular disease.

Dendroaspis natriuretic peptide

Recently, a new member of the natriuretic peptide family, dendroaspis natriuretic peptide (DNP), has been reported. DNP, originally isolated from the venom of *Dendroaspis angusticeps* (green mamba snake), is a 38–amino acid peptide that contains a 17–amino acid disulfide ring structure with a 15-residue C-terminal extension [32]. This peptide, which shares structural similarity to ANP, BNP, and C-type natriuretic peptide, potently vasorelaxes isolated precontracted rodent aorta and canine coronary arteries and augments the formation of cGMP in aortic endothelial and smooth muscle cells [33].

The therapeutic potential of DNP is supported by recent studies in normal animals in which intravenous administration of synthetic DNP had potent natriuretic and diuretic properties that were associated with marked increases in plasma and urinary cGMP [34]. Studies also have reported that DNP has greater affinity for NPRA than ANP or BNP, which may explain its potency [35,36]. In addition, Chen and coworkers [37] have reported that DNP is highly resistant to renal degradation by neutral endopeptidase, which may explain the potency of DNP in mediating cardiorenal actions. In contrast to the other known natriuretic peptides, DNP may have unique characteristics supporting its development as a new intravenous agent for acutely decompensated severe congestive heart failure. It also may have a role as a modulator of cardiac structure and function in the setting of acute myocardial infarction and as a potential oral agent.

Supporting this concept are studies demonstrating in a model of severe heart failure that DNP markedly enhanced renal function including the glomerular filtration rate and sodium excretion together with myocardial unloading and suppression of plasma renin activity [38]. Clinical trials are being planned at the Mayo Clinic to characterize the cardiorenal actions of a DNP-like chimeric peptide as a first step in the clinical development of this new member of the natriuretic peptide family.

Summary

Much progress has occurred since the discovery of ANP. Indeed, the field of natriuretic peptides has moved markedly beyond their role as regulators of renal function. This article has reviewed growing evidence supporting the role of natriuretic peptides as regulators of myocardial structure and function. They are emerging as products not only of the cardiomyocyte but also of the cardiac fibroblast. Studies in vitro and in vivo have clearly established these cardiac hormones as antihypertrophic and antifibrotic. Indications such as cardioprotection for acute myocardial infarction, chronic therapy with oral BNP for hypertension, and next generation DNP-like peptides for acute heart failure may be in the near future. A movement toward such therapeutic strategies in clinical trials in humans with cardiovascular disease is on the horizon.

References

[1] Garbers DL, Chrisman TD, Wiegn P, et al. Membrane guanylyl cyclase receptors: an update. Trends Endocrinol Metab 2006;17(6):251–8.

[2] Cameron VA, Ellmers LJ. Minireview: natriuretic peptides during development of the fetal heart and circulation. Endocrinology 2003;144(6):2191–4.

[3] Lopez MJ, Wong SK, Kishimoto I, et al. Salt-resistant hypertension in mice lacking the guanylyl cyclase-A receptor for atrial natriuretic peptide. Nature 1995;378(6552):65–8.

[4] Oliver PM, Fox JE, Kim R, et al. Hypertension, cardiac hypertrophy, and sudden death in mice lacking natriuretic peptide receptor A. Proc Natl Acad Sci USA 1997;94(26):14730–5.

[5] Holtwick R, van Eickels M, Skryabin BV, et al. Pressure-independent cardiac hypertrophy in mice with cardiomyocyte-restricted inactivation of the atrial natriuretic peptide receptor guanylyl cyclase-A. J Clin Invest 2003;111(9):1399–407.

[6] Lainchbury JG, Burnett JC Jr, Meyer D, et al. Effects of natriuretic peptides on load and myocardial function in normal and heart failure dogs. Am J Physiol Heart Circ Physiol 2000;278(1):H33–40.

[7] Chinkers M, Garbers DL. The protein kinase domain of the ANP receptor is required for signaling. Science 1989;245(4924):1392–4.

[8] Patel JB, Valencik ML, Pritchett AM, et al. Cardiac-specific attenuation of natriuretic peptide A receptor activity accentuates adverse cardiac remodeling and mortality in response to pressure overload. Am J Physiol Heart Circ Physiol 2005;289(2):H777–84.

[9] Tokudome T, Horio T, Kishimoto I, et al. Calcineurin-nuclear factor of activated T cells pathway-dependent cardiac remodeling in mice deficient in guanylyl cyclase A, a receptor for atrial and brain natriuretic peptides. Circulation 2005;111(23): 3095–104.

[10] Silberbach M, Gorenc T, Hershberger RE, et al. Extracellular signal-regulated protein kinase activation is required for the anti-hypertrophic effect of atrial natriuretic factor in neonatal rat ventricular myocytes. J Biol Chem 1999;274(35):24858–64.

[11] Kato T, Muraski J, Chen Y, et al. Atrial natriuretic peptide promotes cardiomyocyte survival by cGMP-dependent nuclear accumulation of zyxin and Akt. J Clin Invest 2005;115(10):2716–30.

[12] Cameron VA, Rademaker MT, Ellmers LJ, et al. Atrial (ANP) and brain natriuretic peptide (BNP) expression after myocardial infarction in sheep: ANP is synthesized by fibroblasts infiltrating the infarct. Endocrinology 2000;141(12):4690–7.

[13] Tsuruda T, Boerrigter G, Huntley BK, et al. Brain natriuretic peptide is produced in cardiac fibroblasts and induces matrix metalloproteinases. Circ Res 2002;91(12):1127–34.

[14] Calderone A, Bel-Hadj S, Drapeau J, et al. Scar myofibroblasts of the infarcted rat heart express natriuretic peptides. J Cell Physiol 2006;207(1): 165–73.

[15] Kapoun AM, Liang F, O'Young G, et al. B-type natriuretic peptide exerts broad functional opposition to transforming growth factor-beta in primary human cardiac fibroblasts: fibrosis, myofibroblast conversion, proliferation, and inflammation. Circ Res 2004;94(4):453–61.

[16] Huntley BK, Sandberg SM, Noser JA, et al. BNP-induced activation of cGMP in human cardiac fibroblasts: interactions with fibronectin and natriuretic peptide receptors. J Cell Physiol 2006;9999:1–7.

[17] Tamura N, Ogawa Y, Chusho H, et al. Cardiac fibrosis in mice lacking brain natriuretic peptide. Proc Natl Acad Sci USA 2000;97(8):4239–44.

[18] Hawkridge AM, Heublein DM, Bergen HR 3rd, et al. Quantitative mass spectral evidence for the absence of circulating brain natriuretic peptide (BNP-32) in severe human heart failure. Proc Natl Acad Sci USA 2005;102(48):17442–7.

[19] Belluardo P, Cataliotti A, Bonaiuto L, et al. Lack of activation of the molecular forms of the BNP system in human grade 1 hypertension and relationship to cardiac hypertrophy. Am J Physiol Heart Circ Physiol 2006;291(4):H1529–35.

[20] Dries DL, Victor RG, Rame JE, et al. Corin gene minor allele defined by 2 missense mutations is common in blacks and associated with high blood pressure and hypertension. Circulation 2005; 112(16):2403–10.

[21] Chan JC, Knudson O, Wu F, et al. Hypertension in mice lacking the proatrial natriuretic peptide convertase corin. Proc Natl Acad Sci USA 2005;102(3): 785–90.

[22] Rubattu S, Bigatti G, Evangelista A, et al. Association of atrial natriuretic peptide and type a natriuretic peptide receptor gene polymorphisms with left ventricular mass in human essential hypertension. J Am Coll Cardiol 2006;48(3):499–505.

[23] Deschepper CF. The many possible benefits of natriuretic peptides after myocardial infarction. Hypertension 2005;46(2):271–2.

[24] Michaels AD, Klein A, Madden JA, et al. Effects of intravenous nesiritide on human coronary vasomotor regulation and myocardial oxygen uptake. Circulation 2003;107(21):2697–701.

[25] Cataliotti A, Boerrigter G, Costello-Boerrigter LC, et al. Brain natriuretic peptide enhances renal actions of furosemide and suppresses furosemide-induced aldosterone activation in experimental heart failure. Circulation 2004;109(13):1680–5.

[26] Ito T, Yoshimura M, Nakamura S, et al. Inhibitory effect of natriuretic peptides on aldosterone synthase gene expression in cultured neonatal rat cardiocytes. Circulation 2003;107(6):807–10.

[27] Brunner-La Rocca HP, Kaye DM, Woods RL, et al. Effects of intravenous brain natriuretic peptide on regional sympathetic activity in patients with chronic heart failure as compared with healthy control subjects. J Am Coll Cardiol 2001;37(5): 1221–7.

[28] Yamahara K, Itoh H, Chun TH, et al. Significance and therapeutic potential of the natriuretic peptides/cGMP/cGMP-dependent protein kinase pathway in vascular regeneration. Proc Natl Acad Sci USA 2003;100(6):3404–9.

[29] Hayashi M, Tsutamoto T, Wada A, et al. Intravenous atrial natriuretic peptide prevents left ventricular remodeling in patients with first anterior acute myocardial infarction. J Am Coll Cardiol 2001; 37(7):1820–6.

[30] Wang W, Ou Y, Shi Y. AlbuBNP, a recombinant B-type natriuretic peptide and human serum albumin fusion hormone, as a long-term therapy of congestive heart failure. Pharm Res 2004;21(11): 2105–11.

[31] Cataliotti A, Schirger JA, Martin FL, et al. Oral human brain natriuretic peptide activates cyclic guanosine 3′,5′-monophosphate and decreases mean arterial pressure. Circulation 2005;112(6):836–40.

[32] Schweitz H, Vigne P, Moinier D, et al. A new member of the natriuretic peptide family is present in the venom of the green mamba (*Dendroaspis angusticeps*). J Biol Chem 1992;267(20):13928–32.

[33] Best PJ, Burnett JC, Wilson SH, et al. Dendroaspis natriuretic peptide relaxes isolated human arteries and veins. Cardiovasc Res 2002;55(2):375–84.

[34] Lisy O, Jougasaki M, Heublein DM, et al. Renal actions of synthetic dendroaspis natriuretic peptide. Kidney Int 1999;56(2):502–8.

[35] Singh G, Kuc RE, Maguire JJ, et al. Novel snake venom ligand dendroaspis natriuretic peptide is selective for natriuretic peptide receptor-A in human heart: downregulation of natriuretic peptide receptor-A in heart failure. Circ Res 2006;99(2):183–90.

[36] Margulies KB, Burnett JC Jr. Visualizing the basis for paracrine natriuretic peptide signaling in human heart. Circ Res 2006;99(2):113–5.

[37] Chen HH, Lainchbury JG, Burnett JC Jr. Natriuretic peptide receptors and neutral endopeptidase in mediating the renal actions of a new therapeutic synthetic natriuretic peptide dendroaspis natriuretic peptide. J Am Coll Cardiol 2002;40(6):1186–91.

[38] Lisy O, Lainchbury JG, Leskinen H, et al. Therapeutic actions of a new synthetic vasoactive and natriuretic peptide, dendroaspis natriuretic peptide, in experimental severe congestive heart failure. Hypertension 2001;37(4):1089–94.

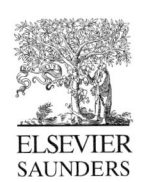

Natriuretic Peptides and Renal Insufficiency: Clinical Significance and Role of Renal Clearance

Benjamin J. Freda, DO[a], Gary S. Francis, MD[b,c],*

[a]*Tufts University School of Medicine, Baystate Medical Center, Springfield, MA, USA*
[b]*Cleveland Clinic, Cleveland, OH, USA*
[c]*Cleveland Clinic Lerner College of Medicine, Case Western Reserve University, Cleveland, OH, USA*

The use of the natriuretic peptides (NPs) BNP and N-terminal proBNP (NT-proBNP) in the diagnosis and management of heart failure (HF) has come at a time of great interest regarding the interrelationship between cardiac and renal dysfunction. As strategies that increase survival in patients who have HF are increasingly used, the clinical importance of limitations imposed by renal dysfunction is becoming more obvious in this patient population [1].

Additionally, there is a substantial burden of HF and asymptomatic structural heart disease in patients who have established chronic kidney disease (CKD) (Table 1) [2]. Reduced renal function as measured by various estimations of the glomerular filtration rate (GFR) is one of the most robust predictors of poor outcomes in patients who have HF [3,4]. Management of the patient who has significant cardiac and renal dysfunction can be difficult [5] and is further complicated by a lack of rigorously tested, evidence-based therapies and underuse of therapies with proven benefit in patients who have preserved renal function [6]. Early and accurate identification of HF in patients who have varying degrees of CKD thus may prove to be an opportunity to provide improved clinical outcomes.

Although originally used to improve the diagnostic accuracy of HF in patients who have acute dyspnea, the role of NPs has evolved greatly over the last few years [7]. Included in this expanded role is the possibility that NPs may be helpful in screening certain asymptomatic populations for the presence of underlying cardiovascular disease (CVD), including HF, left ventricular hypertrophy (LVH), and coronary artery disease (CAD) [8]. Indeed, if screening were to be efficacious, it might be most readily applicable to high-risk patient populations, such as those who have CKD.

Serum levels of BNP and NT-proBNP are commonly elevated in patients who have renal insufficiency. Although it seems reasonable to speculate that elevations in these markers might signify underlying increased cardiac filling pressures, underlying CVD and increased risk for CVD-related adverse events, the impact of renal dysfunction itself as a determinant of serum levels needs to be clarified.

Similarly, the common occurrence of renal insufficiency in patients who have HF mandates a careful consideration of the possible influence of reduced renal function on the production and clearance of NPs from the circulation before the meaning of an elevated serum level is appreciated. This article serves as a review of the role of the kidney in the metabolism and clearance of BNP and NT-proBNP. The clinical usefulness of NP testing is also discussed with attention to diagnostic performance in patients who have HF and concomitant renal dysfunction and patients who have various stages of CKD being evaluated for the presence of CVD and cardiovascular risk.

Cardiovascular disease and renal insufficiency

There is an independent, graded increase in cardiovascular mortality in patients who have

* Corresponding author. Department of Cardiovascular Medicine, Cleveland Clinic, Desk F-25, 9500 Euclid Avenue, Cleveland, OH 44195.
E-mail address: francig@ccf.org (G.S. Francis).

Table 1
Stages of chronic kidney disease[a] according to estimated glomerular filtration rate

Stage	Description	GFR (mL/min)
Stage 1	Kidney damage[a] with normal or elevated GFR	≥90
Stage 2	Kidney damage[a] with mildly reduced GFR	60–89
Stage 3	Moderately reduced GFR	30–59
Stage 4	Severely reduced GFR	15–29
Stage 5	Kidney failure	<15 or dialysis

[a] Chronic kidney disease defined by (1) kidney damage for ≥3 months, defined by pathologic abnormalities or markers of kidney damage (urinary or radiologic abnormalities) or (2). GFR <60 mL/min with or without kidney damage.

Modified from National Kidney Foundation. K/DOQI clinical practice guidelines for chronic kidney disease: evaluation, classification, and stratification. Am J Kidney Dis 2002;39(Suppl 1):S1–266.

progressively severe CKD, with increased risk starting at a GFR of approximately 60 mL/min [9]. The pathophysiology accounting for this relationship is multifactorial and is not fully explained by the presence of traditional risk factors, such as diabetes mellitus and increasing age [10,11]. Furthermore, CAD seems to account for only a small portion of this risk [12].

There is a disproportionate amount of structural heart disease (left ventricular hypertrophy, asymptomatic ventricular dysfunction and CAD) in patients who have CKD [6,13–15]. Estimates from large cross-sectional analyses indicate that as many as 40% of dialysis patients have clinically-defined ischemic heart disease, 40% have HF, and nearly 75% have LVH [14]. Available data indicate that disease prevalence may be similar in patients who have stage 3-4 CKD [15,16]. The presence of LVH is an important predictor of mortality in patients who have CKD, as it is in the general population [17].

In patients who have HF, the prevalence of chronically reduced renal function as defined by contemporary estimates of GFR is likely higher than previously appreciated [18]. In outpatients who have chronic HF, approximately 33% have renal insufficiency as defined by eGFR less than 60 mL/min [19]. In a large database of 52,047 patients who had acutely decompensated HF, 29% had a history of CKD and 20% were admitted with a serum creatinine greater than 2 mg/dL [20].

Natriuretic peptide levels in patients who have chronic kidney disease

Patients who have CKD have higher levels of BNP and NT-proBNP than age- and gender-matched subjects without reduced renal function, even in the absence of clinically apparent HF [21]. It is not surprising that serum levels of NPs increase as renal function diminishes. Several stimuli known to augment NP production, such as increased myocardial wall tension, LVH, and enhanced angiotensin II, increase during the progression of CKD [22,23] (Box 1).

Table 2 illustrates the range of serum levels of BNP and NT-proBNP reported in several recent studies of patients who have varying degrees of renal dysfunction and no evidence of clinical HF. Some asymptomatic patients who have CKD have levels of NPs that are greater than the clinical cut-points used in the diagnosis of acute HF (>100 pg/mL for BNP and >450 pg/mL for NT-proBNP).

Most studies have reported a modest correlation between renal function and NP levels for BNP and NT-proBNP [24,25]. Patients who require dialysis

---

Box 1. Possible determinants of elevated serum natriuretic peptide level in patients who have chronic kidney disease

- Increased myocardial wall tension from hypervolemia, hypertension, or ventricular dysfunction
- Left ventricular hypertrophy
- Reduced renal clearance of natriuretic peptide
- Subclinical ischemia
- Cardiac remodeling/myocardial fibrosis
- Maladaptive neurohormones (ie, angiotensin II)

Table 2
Natriuretic peptide levels in patients who have chronic kidney disease and no clinical suspicion of acute decompensated heart failure

Reference	Assay	Population	Natriuretic peptide levels (mean, pg/mL)		
Defillipe [91]	NT-proBNP (Roche)	CKD predialysis Mean GFR, 33 mL/min	GFR >60 30–59 15–29 <15	149 275 1120 3040	
McCullough [25]	BNP (Biosite)	CKD predialysis Excluded GFR, <15 mL/min	GFR >90 60–89 30–59 15–29	85 132 297 285	
Apple [26]	NT-proBNP (Roche)	Hemodialysis	[a]1st tertile 2nd tertile 3rd tertile >	<4032 4032–18,692 18,692	
Luchner [28]	BNP (Biosite) NT-proBNP (Roche)	CKD predialysis Mean GFR, 71 mL/min	BNP NT-proBNP	75 260	
Lee [102]	BNP (Shionogi)	Hemodialysis	438		
Vickery [92]	BNP (Bayer) NT-proBNP (Roche)	CKD predialysis Mean GFR, 18 mL/min	GFR 30–59 15–29 <15	[b]BNP 31 48 74	[b]NT-proBNP 279 575 1632

[a] Population mean not available; levels reported in tertiles.
[b] Levels reported as population median.

have the highest serum levels of NPs, with measurements that can be greater than several-fold higher than those patients who don not have heart failure [26–28]. One recent study reported that 99% of dialysis patients had elevated NT-proBNP [26]. Limited data suggest that patients receiving peritoneal dialysis also have increased circulating NPs, albeit at lower levels than patients on hemodialysis, despite a similar burden of underlying structural heart disease [29].

Renal role in the clearance of natriuretic peptides

Production of natriuretic peptides

Natriuretic peptides are produced mainly by the heart by way of myocytes [30] and in lesser amounts by cardiac fibroblasts [31]. B-type NPs are synthesized, stored, and released primarily by way of the left ventricle, although other cardiac chambers can also produce these peptides. BNP and NT-proBNP are constitutively released in small amounts by way of the coronary sinus. Increased myocardial wall tension, caused by various signals, leads to a rapid increase in pre-pro BNP mRNA expression [32,33]. The prohormone is metabolized intracellularly to proBNP (1–108 aa), subsequently cleaved by corin, and BNP (1–76) and NT-proBNP (77–108) are released into the circulation in equimolar amounts [34,35].

In vitro studies have demonstrated that renal tubular epithelial cells [36] and glomerular cells [37] may be able to secrete NPs. The clinical significance of this finding is unclear, however.

Metabolism and clearance of natriuretic peptides

Although NT-proBNP and BNP are derived from the same prohormone and are believed to be released in equimolar amounts during myocardial stress, levels of NT-proBNP are higher than BNP in health and disease. Human and animal studies suggest that the elimination half-life for BNP is approximately 3 to 20 minutes [38] and NT-proBNP is approximately 70 minutes [39]. This is contrasted with the t1/2 of ANP, which is much shorter at 3 to 5 minutes. Similar to the B-type NPs, the half-life of NT-proANP is longer than ANP [40]. These observations suggest a difference in metabolism of NPs with a delayed clearance of NT-proBNP compared with BNP.

NPs are primarily metabolized by way of enzymatic degradation by neutral endopeptidases (NEP) and receptor-mediated cellular uptake and lysosomal degradation by way of the neutral peptidase receptor-C (NPR-C) receptor [23]. Animal studies indicate that these mechanisms account for an equal proportion of clearance of BNP [41,42]. Other studies, however, suggest that the relative importance of each mechanism may differ between organs and according to the duration of NP exposure [43–45]. These routes of metabolism are operable within the kidney and other locations throughout the circulation. The NPR-C receptor is located on several tissues, including adrenal gland, kidney, heart, and vascular endothelium [46]. The receptor has a higher affinity for ANP than BNP, possibly explaining the longer half-life and serum level of BNP [47].

The NEP enzymes are located in the peripheral circulation and within several more distinct locations, including the brush border of renal tubular epithelial cells and vascular smooth muscle [48]. NEP metabolizes BNP through degradation of its ring structure [49]. Inhibition of NEP and NPR-C clearance increases the serum levels of BNP [50] but does not have an effect on NT-proBNP levels [35], suggesting an alternate mechanism of clearance for NT-proBNP.

The clearance mechanisms of NT-proBNP are not well described. Although recognition of NP ligand by the NPR-C receptor does not seem to require an intact ring structure [51], it is suggested that structural differences between BNP and NT-proBNP make it unlikely that NT-proBNP is cleared by way of the NPR-C receptor or degraded by way of NEP [39,46].

Because patients who have CKD have greater proportional elevations of NT-proBNP compared with BNP, it has been suggested that glomerular filtration is the principal route of clearance for NT-proBNP [21]. The clearance of BNP also depends on the kidney because of the location of NPR-C receptors and NEP within the nephron. Indeed, there is a similar inverse relationship between GFR and NP level for BNP and NT-proBNP in patients who have preserved or moderately impaired LVEF [25].

It is not clear if the metabolic perturbations of renal failure affect the metabolism of NPs, nor is it clear if uremia per se has an effect on the performance of the commercially available assays used to measure NT-proBNP and BNP. It has been suggested that renal failure could alter peptide metabolism, resulting in different fragment sizes of NPs that are measured to different degrees by individual assays [52]. Although a similar mechanism has been proposed to account for elevated troponin levels in patients who have renal failure [53], it does not seem that currently available assays detect these fragments [54]. Further testing is necessary to clarify the impact of renal failure on peptide metabolism and assay recognition of individual fragments of NPs.

Renal clearance of natriuretic peptides

NT-proBNP and BNP have been measured in the urine of normal control subjects and patients who have HF [55–58]. This is not surprising, considering the small size of the NPs (g3.5–8.5 kDa), relative to other molecules known to be freely filtered across the glomerulus (ie, myoglobin, 18 kDa). In one study, plasma levels of NT-proBNP (1406 ± 1821 pg/mL) were much higher those in the urine (94 ± 31 pg/mL) in patients who have HF. Plasma and urine values, however, were similar in control subjects (36 ± 24 pg/mL versus 67 ± 6 pg/mL) [59].

Recently several human studies have used selective intravenous and intra-arterial catheterization to determine the extraction of BNP and NT-proBNP across several organs, including the kidney [50,60–62]. In a cohort of patients who had essential hypertension, hepatic cirrhosis, and control subjects without kidney or liver disease, concurrent measurements of NT-proBNP and BNP were taken from the renal vein, femoral vein, and femoral artery [60]. Peripheral plasma concentrations did not differ significantly between the groups, and both peptides had an extraction ratio of 0.16 across the kidney. BNP was extracted across the lower limb, however, with an extraction ratio of 0.13, whereas NT-proBNP was not. An earlier report using a different NT-proBNP assay in older patients who had cardiac disease showed a renal extraction ratio similar to those obtained from studies of healthy volunteers [63]. There was some extraction of NT-proBNP across the lower limb, however, suggesting some peripheral, nonrenal metabolism. A similar renal extraction ratio was reported in a cohort of healthy young men using commercially available assays for BNP and NT-proBNP [61].

Tsutamoto recently measured BNP levels in the aorta and coronary sinus in patients who have symptomatic HF and varying degrees of renal dysfunction [62]. BNP production, as measured by the coronary sinus-aorta gradient, related to ejection fraction and left ventricular end diastolic pressure in patients who had and did not have renal dysfunction. Although patients who have renal dysfunction (eGFR <60 mL/min) had higher aortic BNP levels, renal dysfunction was not independently associated with an increase in BNP production. These data suggest that elevations in BNP in patients who have renal dysfunction may be driven more by delayed renal clearance than by increased production.

A recent study suggests that NT-proBNP levels increase to a greater extent compared with BNP in patients who have severe HF and renal dysfunction [64]. Fifteen patients who had end-stage cardiomyopathy had NT-proBNP and BNP measured before and after insertion of a left ventricular assist device. Baseline levels of NT-proBNP and BNP were highly elevated, with NT-proBNP values approximately 10-fold higher than BNP. Both markers were reduced dramatically within 1 week after LVAD implantation, as expected when myocardial wall tension is reduced. The NT-proBNP/BNP ratio increased with eGFR less than 80 mL/min. It is unclear if this was because of greater sensitivity of NT-proBNP in detecting more severe cardiorenal dysfunction or was a result of a greater dependence of NT-proBNP on renal clearance.

Although these studies indicate a similar renal extraction ratio for NT-proBNP and BNP, they do not explain the mechanism of renal clearance (ie, glomerular filtration, tubular secretion, or intrarenal metabolism by NPR-C/NEP), nor do they provide quantitative estimates of the contribution of the kidney to total body clearance of each peptide.

Dialysis-related clearance of natriuretic peptides

Multiple small observational studies using different dialysis membranes and various assays measuring serum levels of BNP and atrial natriuretic peptide (ANP) fragments support the concept that NP levels are reduced to a variable extent during hemodialysis (HD) [65,66]. The relative impact of dialysis clearance versus fluid removal and reduction of cardiac filling pressures, however, is not clear from these studies. Older data with ANP showed that dialysis in the absence of fluid removal (isovolemic dialysis) did not lead to significant changes in plasma ANP levels [67]. NT-proBNP (8.5 kDa) and BNP (3.5 kDa) have a molecular weight less than the size constraint of most high flux dialysis membranes [68], and it is reasonable to expect that some clearance may occur across the dialysis membrane.

There are limited data on the effect of dialysis on BNP and NT-proBNP as measured using current, commercially available assays. One recent study measured BNP and NT-proBNP in dialysate fluid and demonstrated that hemodialysis can clear these peptides from the blood independently from its effect on fluid removal [69]. Serum levels of NT-proBNP and BNP were reduced and peptides were cleared to a similar extent using high flux dialysis membranes. Postdialysis levels remained elevated several-fold higher compared with patients not on dialysis, however, suggesting ongoing stimuli to secretion or low clearance by dialysis.

The impact of clearance by other extracorporeal therapies, including hemodiafiltration and ultrafiltration, remains to be determined. As these therapies have been shown recently to be effective in the management of some patients who have acute decompensated HF [70], further study is required to clarify their effect on NP levels.

Clinical significance of natriuretic peptide testing in patients who have renal insufficiency

Diagnosis of acute heart failure in the presence of renal insufficiency

Recent data indicate that approximately 30% of patients admitted with acute decompensated HF have concomitant renal insufficiency [20]. Diagnostic evaluation of patients who have suspected HF begins with careful assessment for cardinal signs and symptoms, including dyspnea, peripheral edema, and evidence of pulmonary or central congestion. Patients who have acute renal insufficiency or worsening of chronic renal failure can present with similar signs and symptoms, and measurement of renal function is mandatory in all patients being evaluated for possible HF. Natriuretic peptides have been used in evaluation of patients who have dyspnea and have performed better than clinical judgement alone in ruling out a diagnosis of HF [71]. Because both NPs are increased in the presence of renal dysfunction, it is important to evaluate the diagnostic performance of these markers in the presence of renal dysfunction.

The Breathing Not Properly study evaluated the diagnostic performance of a point of care BNP assay in the diagnosis of HF in patients presenting to the emergency department with dyspnea. Patients receiving dialysis or those who had an eGFR less than 15 mL/min were excluded from the study. McCullough and colleagues reported the substudy analysis of 1452 of these patients who had attention to diagnostic performance across a spectrum of renal dysfunction [28].

Estimated GFR was calculated based on the serum creatinine on presentation to the emergency department. The investigators were not able to distinguish acute from chronic renal insufficiency. A total of 432 patients (~30%) had an eGFR of less than 60 mL/min, a value considered to indicate at least moderately reduced renal function. In those patients who had an eGFR less than 60 mL/min and no HF, mean BNP values were 285 to 297 pg/mL. Despite the absence of heart failure, this level is approximately threefold higher than the accepted clinical cut-point used in the diagnosis of HF. Indeed, in those who had varying degrees of renal insufficiency and a BNP value of 100 to 250 pg/mL, 48% to 63% did not have a final diagnosis of HF (Fig. 1). The investigators recommended increasing the cut-point to 200 pg/mL for patients who have an eGFR less than 60 mL/min to maintain optimal diagnostic performance.

In the Pro-BNP Investigation of Dyspnea in the Emergency Department (PRIDE) study, Januzzi and colleagues used NT-proBNP in the evaluation of dyspnea in patients presenting to a single center urban emergency department [72]. Patients who had an Scr greater than 2.5 mg/dL were excluded from the study. NT-proBNP performed well as a diagnostic marker of decompensated HF, with a negative predictive value of 99% at a single cut-point of 300 pg/mL, regardless of age or gender. In a substudy analysis, data were reported on the diagnostic performance of NT-proBNP in patients who had renal insufficiency [27]. In their population, 34% had an eGFR less than 60 mL/min. As with BNP, NT-proBNP levels were generally higher in those who had renal insufficiency. Of those patients who did not have a final diagnosis of HF and a GFR less than 60 mL/min, however, only 36% had NT-proBNP levels greater than the previously published clinical cutpoint. Similar to BNP in the previous study, the test performed well at discriminating HF across the range of reduced GFR (Fig. 1). The investigators recommended that in patients who have an eGFR less than 60 mL/min, the clinical cut-point for NT-proBNP be increased to 1200 pg/mL. At this level, the test performed with 89% sensitivity and 72% specificity.

Similarly, Chenevier-Gobeaux measured NT-proBNP and BNP in patients presenting to the emergency department with dyspnea and renal insufficiency [73]. Although renal insufficiency was associated with higher levels of BNP and NT-proBNP, both markers were able to differentiate cardiac from noncardiac dyspnea across a range of renal dysfunction.

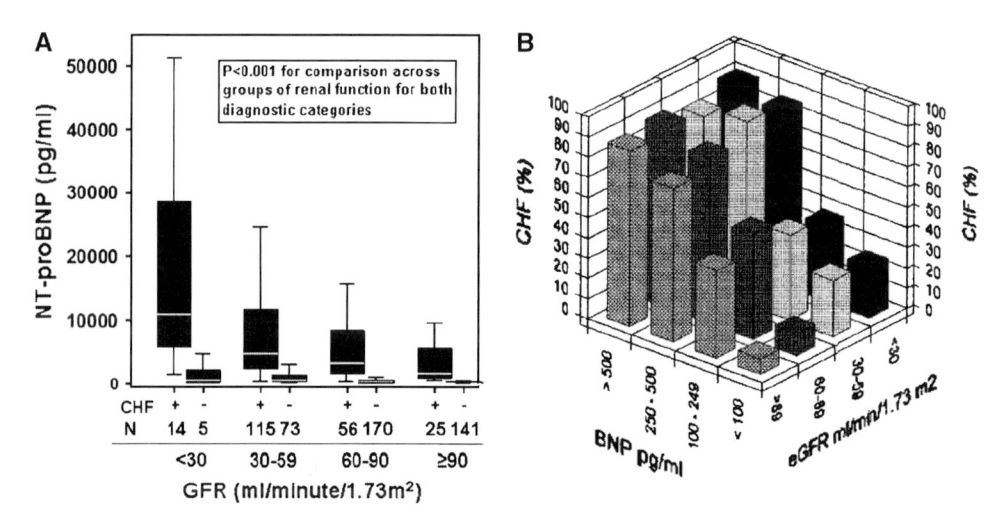

Fig. 1. (A) BNP and NT-proBNP predict the presence of heart failure in patients presenting to the emergency department with dyspnea. (From Anwaruddin S, Lloyd-Jones D, Baggish A, et al. Renal function, congestive heart failure, and amino-terminal natriuretic peptide measurement: results from the ProBNP Investigation of Dyspnea in the Emergency Department (PRIDE) Study. J Am Coll Cardiol 2006;47(1):95; with permission.) (B) Frequency of CHF as the final diagnosis by NKF-KDOQI CKD stage and critical BNP cut points of 100, 250, and 500 pg/mL. To convert BNP in pg/mL to pmol/L, multiply by .289. (From McCullogh PA, Duc P, Omland T, et al. B-type natriuretic peptide and renal function in the diagnosis of heart failure: an analysis from the breathing not properly multinational study. American Journal of Kidney Diseases 2003;41(3):576; with permission. © Copyright 2003 The National Kidney Foundation, Inc.)

Patients who have severely reduced GFR and those receiving dialysis were not included in the aforementioned studies. To the authors' knowledge, there are no data available to assess the performance of BNP and NT-proBNP in the diagnosis of decompensated HF in patients receiving dialysis, and clinicians should not use NP testing for the detection of acute HF in this population.

Natriuretic peptides and prediction of cardiovascular and all-cause mortality

It is estimated that more patients die from cardiovascular disease during the progression of CKD than arrive at dialysis because of advanced renal dysfunction. Multiple serum markers, including cardiac troponins [74], C-reactive protein (CRP) [75], and NPs (see later discussion) have been shown to independently predict cardiovascular and all-cause mortality in patients who have varying degrees of renal impairment.

Zoccali and colleagues studied 246 patients on hemo- and peritoneal dialysis who did not have clinical HF and who had an ejection fraction greater than 35% [76]. Baseline echocardiograms and NP levels were measured using older assay techniques. Patients were followed for 2 years. NP levels were highest in patients who had increased LV mass or reduced systolic function. BNP and ANP were independently predictive of ejection fraction and LV mass. Only BNP, however, was independently predictive of cardiovascular or all-cause death, even after adjustment for LV mass and ejection fraction. BNP was also independently predictive of cardiac death in a study of 164 patients on hemodialysis [66]. When BNP was entered into a multivariate model, however, relative risk for mortality was lower than that predicted by CRP or LV mass.

A panel of biomarkers, including NT-proBNP, troponin T (TnT), troponin I (TnI), and CRP were studied in a cohort of 399 patients who had end-stage renal disease (ESRD) and no clinical HF [26]. Cardiac troponin and CRP were highly predictive of all-cause mortality at currently defined clinical cut-points used in patients who did not have renal dysfunction. NT-proBNP levels were universally elevated (middle tertile, 4032–18,693 pg/mL) with 99% of patients having levels higher than accepted clinical cut-points. Using tertile analysis, however, NT-proBNP was predictive of survival at 1 and 2 years follow-up (Fig. 2).

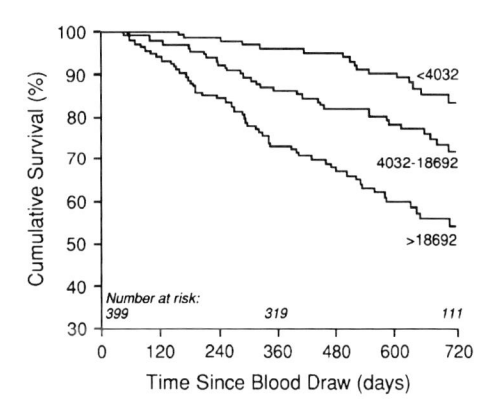

Fig. 2. NT-proBNP predicts mortality in patients on hemodialysis. Kap2lan-Meier survival cures by baseline NT-proBNP tertiles. The total numbers of patients at risk at baseline and after 1 and 2 years are shown at the bottom of the graph. (*From* Apple FS, Murakami MM, Pearce LA, et al. Multi-biomarker risk stratification of N-terminal pro-B-type natriuretic peptide, high-sensitivity C-reactive protein, and cardiac troponin T and I in end-stage renal disease for all-cause death. Clin Chem 2004;50(12):2281; with permission.)

There are fewer data available on the prognostic significance of NPs in patients who have nondialysis-dependent, less severe forms of CKD. Takami and colleagues studied 103 patients who had CKD, EF greater than 40%, and no clinical HF [77]. Patients had severe CKD with a mean CrCl of 15±1 mL/min. BNP levels were elevated compared with hypertensive control subjects who had normal renal function. In patients who had CKD, BNP levels were 71 ± 9 and 257 ± 39 pg/mL, in the groups with and without echocardiographic evidence of LV overload, respectively. Although mortality was not an endpoint, BNP was an independent predictor of the development of congestive heart failure (CHF) requiring admission. BNP had a positive predictive value of 86.7% but a sensitivity of only 52% for predicting HF admission using a cut-point of 150 pg/mL.

More recently Carr and colleagues reported the prognostic ability of NT-proBNP in a cohort of patients who had CKD and no history or clinical evidence of HF [78]. Patients had a median Scr of approximately 2.6 mg/dL and a median NT-proBNP of 291 pmol/L. In patients who had an Scr greater than the median, an NT-proBNP level greater than 355 pmol/L was predictive of all-cause mortality with a sensitivity of 100% and a specificity of 65.8% (Fig. 3).

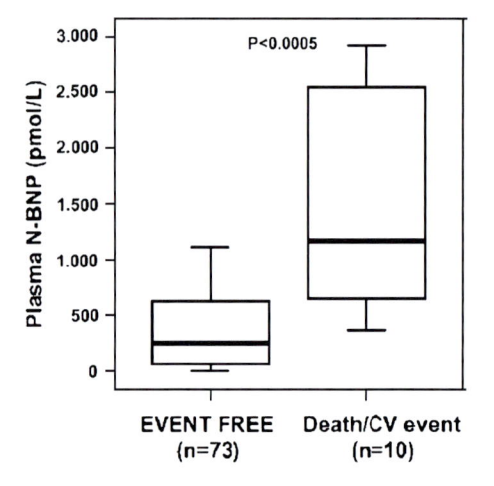

Fig. 3. NT-proBNP levels are elevated in patients who have nondialysis-dependent CKD and death or new CV event. (*From* Carr SJ, Bavanandan S, Fentum B, et al. Prognostic potential of brain natriuretic peptide (BNP) in predialysis chronic kidney disease. Clin Sci 2005;109(1):79; with permission.)

NT-proBNP was also independently predictive of survival in a cohort of patients who had acutely decompensated HF and an eGFR less than 60 mL/min [27]. To clarify the significance of these initial observations and provide clinicians with optimal clinical cut-points to estimate mortality risk, larger series of patients across a greater spectrum of renal dysfunction are required.

Natriuretic peptides as markers of cardiovascular disease

The true prevalence of CVD in patients who have CKD has been estimated from larger cross-sectional studies but remains to be determined more precisely. In this population, CVD encompasses a broad range of pathologies, including LVH, diastolic and systolic dysfunction, ischemic heart disease, and peripheral arteriosclerosis. Some have speculated that patients who have CKD may develop a form of myocardial injury referred to as uremic cardiomyopathy, characterized by myocyte disarray and fibrosis [79] (Fig. 4). Not surprisingly, limited data suggest the degree of fibrosis has important prognostic significance [80]. It is tempting to speculate that NPs may act as a marker of underlying myocardial fibrosis in patients who have CKD [31].

Because many patients remain asymptomatic until CVD is advanced and structural changes are well established [81], it may be reasonable to speculate that early identification of CVD could prove beneficial in patients who have CKD [82]. Indeed, once clinical HF is manifest, survival is dramatically reduced in patients who have severe CKD, with only approximately 33% of patients still alive at 2 years [83]. Studies using cardiac troponin T indicate that it is possible for a cardiac biomarker to predict the presence of underlying CVD in asymptomatic patients who have various degrees of CKD [74,84].

In patients who do not have CKD or clinically apparent HF, NP levels are higher in the presence of LVH, CAD, and ventricular dysfunction [23,85]. Furthermore, NP levels are predictive of overall cardiovascular morbidity and mortality in patients who do not have apparent CKD or HF [86,87].

Early studies in patients receiving dialysis suggest that elevations of BNP are driven by the

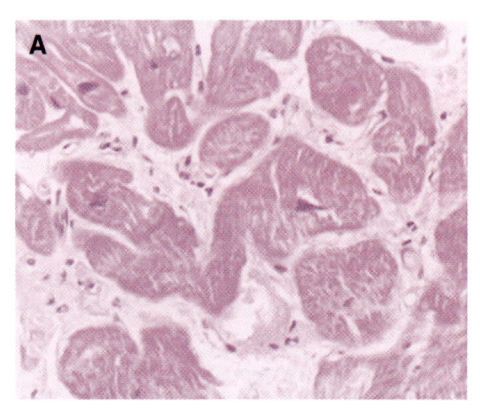

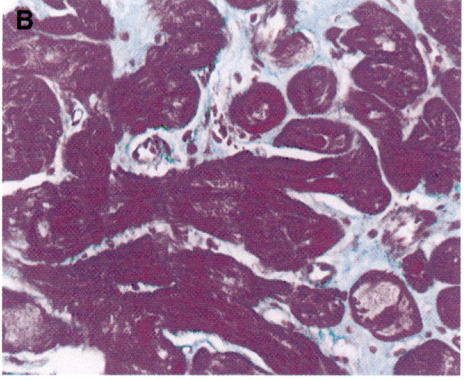

Fig. 4. Myocardial hypertrophy and fibrosis in uremic cardiomyopathy. (*From* Aoki J, Ikari Y, Nakajima H, et al. Clinical and pathologic characteristics of dilated cardiomyopathy in hemodialysis patients. Kidney Int 2005;67(1):336; with permission.)

underlying presence of LVH [88]. In a small subgroup, patients who had ESRD and no underlying LVH, left ventricular dysfunction, previous MI, CAD, stroke, diabetes, or hypertension, levels of BNP were not significantly different from those in patients who have preserved renal function.

Similarly, in a group of patients who had severe nondialysis-dependent CKD (mean Scr, 4.9), echocardiographic markers of LV overload and diastolic dysfunction were independent determinants of BNP levels, even after adjustment for renal dysfunction [77]. In patients receiving hemodialysis without overt HF, BNP was useful for indicating the presence of underlying LVH and LV systolic dysfunction as measured by echocardiography [89]. Serum levels of BNP correlated with pulmonary artery wedge pressure and LVEF in a small group of patients who had CAD on chronic maintenance dialysis [90].

Recent studies using more contemporary assays suggest that BNP and NT-proBNP may predict the presence of underlying CVD in patients who have varying degrees of CKD. In a cohort of 207 ambulatory, asymptomatic patients who had a mean eGFR of 33 mL/min, NT-proBNP levels were independently predictive of LVH and prior CAD events [91]. In a subset of patients who underwent echocardiography, NT-proBNP correlated significantly with prior CAD independent of the presence of underlying LVH. Diagnostic performance was modest at a cut-point of 318 pg/mL, with a sensitivity of 78% and a specificity of 56%. It is not clear whether NT-proBNP was predicting the presence of underlying CAD or whether patients who already had established CAD events had elevated NT-proBNP levels. A similar study concluded that LV mass was an independent predictor of BNP and NT-proBNP levels in 213 predialysis patients who had a median eGFR of 18 mL/min [92].

A recent cross-sectional study of patients who had CKD, including patients on hemodialysis and those with functioning renal allografts, analyzed the relationship between BNP levels and echocardiographically-determined LV dysfunction, including LVH [93]. Patients who had DM and known CAD were excluded. BNP predicted the presence of LVH or LV systolic dysfunction with a sensitivity of 61% and 72%, respectively. Specificity was low, however, in the range of 40% to 67%, and when GFR was included in the multivariate analysis, LV systolic dysfunction was not an independent predictor of BNP.

Although NT-proBNP and BNP seem to predict risk and some aspects of underlying CVD, data are lacking on the usefulness of a strategy that incorporates their use into clinical decision making. Such a strategy, however, may prove most useful at early stages of CKD before CVD becomes well established. Such a strategy may identify patients who merit further testing with echocardiography and consideration for therapies that may be effective even in patients who have severe CKD [94–97]. Additionally, information garnered from NP measurement may help clinicians decide on appropriate cardiac evaluation and treatment in patients being evaluated for renal transplantation and individualization of dialysis prescription to reduce cardiac load [98–100].

Estimation of hydration status in patients on dialysis

The determination of hydration status is complex in patients receiving dialysis, and a gold standard that is readily accessible as a measure of extracellular fluid is not yet available [101]. Inadequate control of volume can result in further cardiac strain and progression of CVD, whereas overly aggressive volume removal can precipitate hemodynamic instability.

Natriuretic peptides increase in hypervolemic states, and thus have been investigated as a marker of hydration status in patients receiving hemodialysis. Using ultrasonic measurements of inferior vena cava diameter and bioimpedance measures of extracellular fluid as a means to quantify volume status, Lee and colleagues reported the relationship between BNP levels and hydration status in 49 dialysis patients [102]. BNP levels did not change during dialysis; however, pre- and post-HD values were significantly higher in overhydrated (716 ± 576 and 770 ± 619 pg/mL) patients compared with those deemed euvolemic (229 ± 203 and 224 ± 176 pg/mL). BNP was unable to predict a difference between euvolemic and under-hydrated patients, although the number of under-hydrated patients was small.

Fagugli and colleagues demonstrated that BNP levels were associated with hydration status as measured by bioimpedance in a group of dialysis patients who did not have known LV dysfunction [103]. Fewer data are available in peritoneal dialysis patients, but a recent report suggests that although NT-proBNP levels are closely associated with LV mass and systolic function in patients on peritoneal dialysis, they are not as closely linked with hydration status as measured by bioimpedance [104].

Natriuretic peptides have been used to monitor HF therapy in populations without reduced renal function, though few data are available [105] and some are forthcoming [106]. Similar studies should be performed in patients receiving dialytic therapies in an effort to determine if NP testing could optimize the dialysis prescription and fluid balance, resulting in improvement in cardiovascular outcomes. Ideally these studies should be performed before NP testing is incorporated into the routine care of patients being treated with chronic dialysis.

It is likely that elevated NP levels reflect a multitude of stimuli in patients on dialysis. Reduced renal clearance, underlying left ventricular hypertrophy, left ventricular dysfunction, subclinical ischemia, and persistent hypervolemia all contribute to the development of an elevated NP level in this population. Natriuretic peptide levels likely provide a measure of overall cardiac load rather than a pure surrogate marker of the patient's current volume status. The intra-individual biologic variation of NPs, superimposed on individual dialysis schedules, should be studied before a strategy using these markers is adopted into clinical practice.

Summary

The use of NPs for diagnosis and prognosis of CVD comes at a time of great interest pertaining to the important interaction between cardiac and renal dysfunction. Although it is clear that BNP and NT-proBNP are metabolized by the kidney and their levels are increased in patients who have renal dysfunction even in the absence of clinical HF, a precise understanding of their metabolic pathways is not clear at this time. Current data indicate that there are important differences in metabolism and clearance of BNP and NT-proBNP. Although BNP and NT-proBNP perform reasonably well in the diagnosis of acute heart failure in patients who have concomitant renal insufficiency (eGFR <60 mL/min) being evaluated for acute dyspnea, both markers require an adjustment in the clinical cut-point greater than the accepted levels used for patients who have preserved renal function.

Even less is known regarding the diagnostic performance of these markers in the acute setting in patients who have more severe CKD and ESRD. Clinicians caring for patients who have ESRD should not use NPs to reliably predict or rule out the presence of underlying ventricular dysfunction. Further testing is required in patients who have less severe forms of CKD to ascertain whether NP levels can serve as markers of clinically important cardiac disease before symptoms or geometric changes of the LV occur. Although NP levels correlate with underlying heart disease and mortality in patients receiving dialysis, current data do not support the use of these markers as a surrogate marker of volume status.

References

[1] Shlipak MG, Massie BM. The clinical challenge of cardiorenal syndrome. Circulation 2004;110(12): 1514–7.

[2] National Kidney Foundation. K/DOQI clinical practice guidelines for chronic kidney disease: evaluation, classification, and stratification. Am J Kidney Dis 2002;39(Suppl 1):S1–266.

[3] Bart BA, Goldsmith SR. Aggravated renal dysfunction and the acute management of advanced chronic heart failure. Am Heart J 1999;138:200–2.

[4] Hillege HL, et al. Renal function, neurohormonal activation, and survival in patients with chronic heart failure. Circulation 2000;102:203–10.

[5] Shlipak MG. Pharmacotherapy for heart failure in patients with renal insufficiency. Ann Intern Med 2003;138:917–24.

[6] Culleton BF, Hemmelgarn B. Inadequate treatment of cardiovascular disease and cardiovascular disease risk factors in dialysis patients: a commentary. Semin Dial 2004;17:342–5.

[7] Weber M, Hamm C. Role of B-type natriuretic peptide (BNP) and NT-proBNP in clinical routine. Heart 2006;92:843–9.

[8] Kragelund C, et al. Biochemical cardiac risk markers in the general population, hypertension and coronary artery disease. Scand J Clin Lab Invest Suppl 2005;240:138–42.

[9] Go AS, et al. Chronic kidney disease and the risks of death, cardiovascular events, and hospitalization. N Engl J Med 2004;351:1296–305.

[10] Ritz E, McClellan WM. Overview: increased cardiovascular risk in patients with minor renal dysfunction: an emerging issue with far-reaching consequences. J Am Soc Nephrol 2004;15:513–6.

[11] Varma R, et al. Chronic renal dysfunction as an independent risk factor for the development of cardiovascular disease. Cardiol Rev 2005;13:98–107.

[12] Stack AG, Bloembergen WE. Prevalence and clinical correlates of coronary artery disease among new dialysis patients in the United States:

a cross-sectional study. J Am Soc Nephrol 2001;12: 1516–23.
[13] Levin A, et al. Left ventricular mass index increase in early renal disease: impact of decline in hemoglobin. Am J Kidney Dis 1999;34:125–34.
[14] Sarnak MJ, et al. Kidney disease as a risk factor for development of cardiovascular disease: a statement from the American Heart Association Councils on Kidney in Cardiovascular Disease, High Blood Pressure Research, Clinical Cardiology, and Epidemiology and Prevention. Hypertension 2003;42: 1050–65.
[15] Levin A. Clinical epidemiology of cardiovascular disease in chronic kidney disease prior to dialysis. Semin Dial 2003;16:101–5.
[16] Muntner P, et al. Renal insufficiency and subsequent death resulting from cardiovascular disease in the United States. J Am Soc Nephrol 2002;13: 745–53.
[17] Haider AW, et al. Increased left ventricular mass and hypertrophy are associated with increased risk for sudden death. J Am Coll Cardiol 1998;32: 1454–9.
[18] Smith GL, et al. Renal impairment and outcomes in heart failure: systematic review and meta-analysis. J Am Coll Cardiol 2006;47:1987–96.
[19] Dries DL, et al. The prognostic implications of renal insufficiency in asymptomatic and symptomatic patients with left ventricular systolic dysfunction. J Am Coll Cardiol 2000;35:681–9.
[20] Fonarow GC. The Acute Decompensated Heart Failure National Registry (ADHERE): opportunities to improve care of patients hospitalized with acute decompensated heart failure. Rev Cardiovasc Med 2003;4(Suppl 7):S21–30.
[21] McCullough PA, Sandberg KR. Sorting out the evidence on natriuretic peptides. Rev Cardiovasc Med 2003;4(Suppl 4):S13–9.
[22] Focaccio A, et al. Angiotensin II directly stimulates release of atrial natriuretic factor in isolated rabbit hearts. Circulation 1993;87:192–8.
[23] Munagala VK, Burnett J, John C, et al. The natriuretic peptides in cardiovascular medicine. Curr Probl Cardiol 2004;29:707–69.
[24] Richards M, et al. Comparison of B-type natriuretic peptides for assessment of cardiac function and prognosis in stable ischemic heart disease. J Am Coll Cardiol 2006;47:52–60.
[25] Luchner A, et al. Effect of compensated renal dysfunction on approved heart failure markers: direct comparison of brain natriuretic peptide (BNP) and N-terminal pro-BNP. Hypertension 2005;46:118–23.
[26] Apple FS, et al. Multi-biomarker risk stratification of N-terminal pro-B-type natriuretic peptide, high-sensitivity C-reactive protein, and cardiac troponin T and I in end-stage renal disease for all-cause death. Clin Chem 2004;50:2279–85.

[27] Anwaruddin S, et al. Renal function, congestive heart failure, and amino-terminal pro-brain natriuretic peptide measurement: results from the ProBNP Investigation of Dyspnea in the Emergency Department (PRIDE) Study. J Am Coll Cardiol 2006;47:91–7.
[28] McCullough PA, et al. B-type natriuretic peptide and renal function in the diagnosis of heart failure: an analysis from the breathing not properly multinational study. Am J Kidney Dis 2003;41: 571–9.
[29] Taskapan MC, et al. Brain natriuretic peptide and its relationship to left ventricular hypertrophy in patients on peritoneal dialysis or hemodialysis less than 3 years. Ren Fail 2006;28:133–9.
[30] Yasue H, et al. Localization and mechanism of secretion of B-type natriuretic peptide in comparison with those of A-type natriuretic peptide in normal subjects and patients with heart failure. Circulation 1994;90:195–203.
[31] Tsuruda T, et al. Brain natriuretic peptide is produced in cardiac fibroblasts and induces matrix metalloproteinases. Circ Res 2002;91:1127–34.
[32] Ma KK, Banas K, de Bold AJ. Determinants of inducible brain natriuretic peptide promoter activity. Regul Pept 2005;128:169–76.
[33] Nakagawa O, et al. Rapid transcriptional activation and early mRNA turnover of brain natriuretic peptide in cardiocyte hypertrophy. Evidence for brain natriuretic peptide as an "emergency" cardiac hormone against ventricular overload. J Clin Invest 1995;96(3):1280–7.
[34] Ruskoaho H. Cardiac hormones as diagnostic tools in heart failure. Endocr Rev 2003;24:341–56.
[35] Pemberton CJ, et al. Amino-terminal proBNP in ovine plasma: evidence for enhanced secretion in response to cardiac overload. Am J Physiol Heart Circ Physiol 1998;275:H1200–8.
[36] Mistry SK, et al. Differential expression and synthesis of natriuretic peptides determines natriuretic peptide receptor expression in primary cultures of human proximal tubular cells. J Hypertens 2001;19:255–62.
[37] Lai KN, et al. Gene expression and synthesis of natriuretic peptides by cultured human glomerular cells. J Hypertens 1999;17:575–83.
[38] McGregor A, et al. Brain natriuretic peptide administered to man: actions and metabolism. J Clin Endocrinol Metab 1990;70:1103–7.
[39] Pemberton CJ, et al. Deconvolution analysis of cardiac natriuretic peptides during acute volume overload. Hypertension 2000;36:355–9.
[40] Thibault G, et al. NH2-terminal fragment of rat pro-atrial natriuretic factor in the circulation: Identification, radioimmunoassay and half-life. Peptides 1988;9:47–53.
[41] Rademaker MT, et al. Clearance receptors and endopeptidase: equal role in natriuretic peptide

metabolism in heart failure. Am J Physiol Heart Circ Physiol 1997;273:H2372–9.
[42] Charles CJ, et al. Clearance receptors and endopeptidase 24.11: equal role in natriuretic peptide metabolism in conscious sheep. Am J Physiol Regul Integr Comp Physiol 1996;271:R373–80.
[43] Kishimoto I, et al. Downregulation of C-receptor by natriuretic peptides by way of ANP-B receptor in vascular smooth muscle cells. Am J Physiol Heart Circ Physiol 1993;265:H1373–9.
[44] Smith M, et al. Delayed metabolism of human brain natriuretic peptide reflects resistance to neutral endopeptidase. J Endocrinol 2000;167:239–46.
[45] Walther T, et al. Biochemical analysis of neutral endopeptidase activity reveals independent catabolism of atrial and brain natriuretic peptide. Biol Chem 2004;385:179–84.
[46] Vanderheyden M, Bartunek J, Goethals M. Brain and other natriuretic peptides: molecular aspects. Eur J Heart Fail 2004;6:261–8.
[47] Suga S-I, et al. Receptor selectivity of natriuretic peptide family, atrial natriuretic peptide, brain natriuretic peptide, and C-type natriuretic peptide. Endocrinology 1992;130:229–39.
[48] Schulz WW, et al. Ultrastructural localization of angiotensin I-converting enzyme (EC 3.4.15.1) and neutral metalloendopeptidase (EC 3.4.24.11) in the proximal tubule of the human kidney. Lab Invest 1988;59:789–97.
[49] Kenny AJ, Bourne A, Ingram J. Hydrolysis of human and pig brain natriuretic peptides, urodilatin, C-type natriuretic peptide and some C-receptor ligands by endopeptidase-24.11. Biochem J 1993;291:83–8.
[50] Lainchbury JG, et al. Regional plasma levels of cardiac peptides and their response to acute neutral endopeptidase inhibition in man. Clin Sci (Lond) 1998;95:547–55.
[51] Maack T. The broad homeostatic role of natriuretic peptides. Arq Bras Endocrinol Metabol 2006;50:198–207.
[52] Jaffe AS, Apple FS, Babuin L. Why We don't know the answer may be more important than the specific question. Clin Chem 2004;50:1495–7.
[53] Diris JH, et al. Impaired renal clearance explains elevated troponin T fragments in hemodialysis patients. Circulation 2004;109:23–5.
[54] Fahie-Wilson MN, et al. Cardiac troponin T circulates in the free, intact form in patients with kidney failure. Clin Chem 2006;52:414–20.
[55] Togashi K, Fujita S, Kawakami M. Presence of brain natriuretic peptide in urine. Clin Chem 1992;38:322–3.
[56] Ng LL, et al. Diagnosis of heart failure using urinary natriuretic peptides. Clin Sci (Lond) 2004;106:129–33.
[57] Ng LL, et al. Community screening for left ventricular systolic dysfunction using plasma and urinary natriuretic peptides. J Am Coll Cardiol 2005;45:1043–50.
[58] Heringlake M, et al. Effects of tilting and volume loading on plasma levels and urinary excretion of relaxin, NT-pro-ANP, and NT-pro-BNP in male volunteers. J Appl Physiol 2004;97:173–9.
[59] Cortes R, et al. Diagnostic and prognostic value of urine NT-proBNP levels in heart failure patients. Eur J Heart Fail 2006;21:2507–12.
[60] Goetze JP, et al. BNP and N-terminal proBNP are both extracted in the normal kidney. Eur J Clin Invest 2006;36:8–15.
[61] Schou M, et al. Kidneys extract BNP and NT-proBNP in healthy young men. J Appl Physiol 2005;99:1676–80.
[62] Tsutamoto T, et al. Relationship between renal function and plasma brain natriuretic peptide in patients with heart failure. J Am Coll Cardiol 2006;47:582–6.
[63] Hunt PJ, et al. Immunoreactive amino-terminal pro-brain natriuretic peptide (NT-PROBNP): a new marker of cardiac impairment. Clin Endocrinol (Oxf) 1997;47:287–96.
[64] Kemperman H, et al. B-type natriuretic peptide (BNP) and N-terminal proBNP in patients with end-stage heart failure supported by a left ventricular assist device. Clin Chem 2004;50:1670–2.
[65] Suresh M, Farrington K. Natriuretic peptides and the dialysis patient. Semin Dial 2005;18:409–19.
[66] Naganuma T, et al. The prognostic role of brain natriuretic peptides in hemodialysis patients. Am J Nephrol 2002;22:437–44.
[67] Tsuchiya K, Sanaka T, Ando A. Renal and hemodynamic effects of synthetic atrial natriuretic peptide in dogs with chronic renal failure. Nippon Jinzo Gakkai Shi 1989;31:151–7.
[68] Mehta RL. Continuous renal replacement therapy in the critically ill patient. Kidney Int 2005;67:781–95.
[69] Wahl HG, et al. Elimination of the cardiac natriuretic peptides B-type natriuretic peptide (BNP) and N-terminal proBNP by hemodialysis. Clin Chem 2004;50:1071–4.
[70] Boyle A. Ultrafiltration for acute decompensated heart failure. Expert Rev Med Devices 2005;2:689–97.
[71] McCullough PA, et al. B-type natriuretic peptide and clinical judgment in emergency diagnosis of heart failure: analysis from Breathing Not Properly (BNP) Multinational Study. Circulation 2002;106(4):416–22.
[72] Januzzi JL Jr, et al. The N-terminal Pro-BNP investigation of dyspnea in the emergency department (PRIDE) study. Am J Cardiol 2005;95:948–54.
[73] Chenevier-Gobeaux C, et al. Influence of renal function on N-terminal pro-brain natriuretic peptide (NT-proBNP) in patients admitted for dyspnoea in the Emergency Department: comparison

with brain natriuretic peptide (BNP). Clin Chim Acta 2005;361:167–75.
[74] Freda BJ, et al. Cardiac troponins in renal insufficiency: review and clinical implications. J Am Coll Cardiol 2002;40:2065–71.
[75] Zoccali C. Biomarkers in chronic kidney disease: utility and issues towards better understanding. Curr Opin Nephrol Hypertens 2005;14:532–7.
[76] Zoccali C, et al. Cardiac natriuretic peptides are related to left ventricular mass and function and predict mortality in dialysis patients. J Am Soc Nephrol 2001;12:1508–15.
[77] Takami Y, et al. Diagnostic and prognostic value of plasma brain natriuretic peptide in non-dialysis-dependent CRF. Am J Kidney Dis 2004;44:420–8.
[78] Carr SJ, et al. Prognostic potential of brain natriuretic peptide (BNP) in predialysis chronic kidney disease patients. Clin Sci (Lond) 2005;109:75–82.
[79] Amann K, Ritz E. Reduced cardiac ischaemia tolerance in uraemia—what is the role of structural abnormalities of the heart? Nephrol Dial Transplant 1996;11:1238–41.
[80] Aoki J, et al. Clinical and pathologic characteristics of dilated cardiomyopathy in hemodialysis patients. Kidney Int 2005;67:333–40.
[81] Ohtake T, et al. High prevalence of occult coronary artery stenosis in patients with chronic kidney disease at the initiation of renal replacement therapy: an angiographic examination. J Am Soc Nephrol 2005;16:1141–8.
[82] No authors. Effect of enalapril on mortality and the development of heart failure in asymptomatic patients with reduced left ventricular ejection fractions. The SOLVD Investigators. N Engl J Med 1992;327:685–91.
[83] Parfrey PS, Harnett JD, Barre PE. The natural history of myocardial disease in dialysis patients. J Am Soc Nephrol 1991;2:2–12.
[84] deFilippi C, et al. Cardiac troponin T and C-reactive protein for predicting prognosis, coronary atherosclerosis, and cardiomyopathy in patients undergoing long-term hemodialysis. JAMA 2003;290:353–9.
[85] Weber M, et al. N-terminal B-type natriuretic peptide predicts extent of coronary artery disease and ischemia in patients with stable angina pectoris. Am Heart J 2004;148:612–20.
[86] Kistorp C, et al. N-terminal pro-brain natriuretic peptide, C-reactive protein, and urinary albumin levels as predictors of mortality and cardiovascular events in older adults. JAMA 2005;293:1609–16.
[87] Kragelund C, et al. N-terminal pro-B-type natriuretic peptide and long-term mortality in stable coronary heart disease. N Engl J Med 2005;352:666–75.
[88] Cataliotti A, et al. Circulating natriuretic peptide concentrations in patients with end-stage renal disease: role of brain natriuretic peptide as a biomarker for ventricular remodeling. Mayo Clin Proc 2001;76:1111–9.

[89] Mallamaci F, et al. Diagnostic potential of cardiac natriuretic peptides in dialysis patients. Kidney Int 2001;59:1559–66.
[90] Osajima A, et al. Comparison of plasma levels of mature adrenomedullin and natriuretic peptide as markers of cardiac function in hemodialysis patients with coronary artery disease. Nephron 2002;92:832–9.
[91] deFilippi, et al. N-terminal pro-B-type natriuretic peptide for predicting coronary disease and left ventricular hypertrophy in asymptomatic CKD not requiring dialysis. Am J Kidney Dis 2005;46:35–44.
[92] Vickery, et al. B-type natriuretic peptide (BNP) and amino-terminal proBNP in patients with CKD: relationship to renal function and left ventricular hypertrophy. Am J Kidney Dis 2005;46:610–20.
[93] Mark PB, et al. Diagnostic potential of circulating natriuretic peptides in chronic kidney disease. Nephrol Dial Transplant 2006;21:402–10.
[94] Yu WC, et al. Effect of ramipril on left ventricular mass in normotensive hemodialysis patients. Am J Kidney Dis 2006;47:478–84.
[95] Cice G, et al. Dilated cardiomyopathy in dialysis patients–beneficial effects of carvedilol: a double-blind, placebo-controlled trial. J Am Coll Cardiol 2001;37:407–11.
[96] Takahashi A, Takase H, Toriyama T, et al. Candesartan, an angiotensin II type-1 receptor blocker, reduces cardiovascular events in patients on chronic haemodialysis—a randomized study. Nephrol Dial Transplant 2006;21(9):2507–12.
[97] Efrati S, et al. ACE inhibitors and survival of hemodialysis patients. Am J Kidney Dis 2002;40:1023–9.
[98] Cheung AK, et al. Cardiac diseases in maintenance hemodialysis patients. Results of the HEMO Study 2004;65:2380–9.
[99] Dastoor H, et al. Plasma BNP in patients on maintenance haemodialysis: a guide to management? J Hypertens 2005;23:23–8.
[100] Rigatto C, et al. Congestive heart failure in renal transplant recipients: risk factors, outcomes, and relationship with ischemic heart disease. J Am Soc Nephrol 2002;13:1084–90.
[101] Ishibe S, Peixoto AJ. Methods of assessment of volume status and intercompartmental fluid shifts in hemodialysis patients: implications in clinical practice. Semin Dial 2004;17:37–43.
[102] Lee SW, et al. Plasma brain natriuretic peptide concentration on assessment of hydration status in hemodialysis patient. Am J Kidney Dis 2003;41:1257–66.
[103] Fagugli RM, et al. Association between brain natriuretic peptide and extracellular water in hemodialysis patients. Nephron Clin Pract 2003;95:c60–6.
[104] Lee JA, et al. Association between serum n-terminal pro-brain natriuretic peptide concentration

and left ventricular dysfunction and extracellular water in continuous ambulatory peritoneal dialysis patients. Perit Dial Int 2006;26:360–5.

[105] Troughton RW, et al. Treatment of heart failure guided by plasma aminoterminal brain natriuretic peptide (N-BNP) concentrations. Lancet 2000; 355:1126–30.

[106] Shah MR, et al. Testing new targets of therapy in advanced heart failure: the design and rationale of the Strategies for Tailoring Advanced Heart Failure Regimens in the Outpatient Setting: BRain NatrIuretic Peptide Versus the Clinical Conges-Tion ScorE (STARBRITE) trial. Am Heart J 2005;150:893–8.

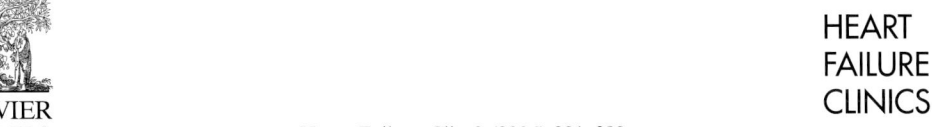

Plasma BNP/NT-proBNP Assays: What Do They Target and What Else Might They Recognize?

Alan H.B. Wu, PhD[a,b,*]

[a]University of California, San Francisco, CA, USA
[b]San Francisco General Hospital, San Francisco, CA, USA

Commercial assays for B-type natriuretic peptide and the amino-terminus NT-proBNP have been cleared by the U.S. Food and Drug Administration (FDA) and are now widely used biomarkers for heart failure diagnosis, staging, and risk stratification for future adverse events. Increased concentrations of BNP and NT-proBNP are also predictive for cardiovascular deaths for patients who present with acute coronary syndromes, and some commercial assays have received clearance for this indication also. In the future, results of BNP and NT-proBNP testing may be important in monitoring outpatient drug therapy of heart failure patients and for screening for left ventricular dysfunction in patients who are asymptomatic for heart failure. None of the commercial assays have clearance for these latter indications to date, however.

Release and stability of natriuretic peptide forms in human blood

The secretion of BNP and NT-proBNP from the precursor molecule proBNP has been well studied and is discussed elsewhere in this issue by Ramos and de Bold. A summary of this relationship is shown in Fig. 1. BNP (amino acids 77–108) and NT-proBNP (amino acids 1–76) are derived from proBNP (amino acids 1–108). Once released into blood, BNP (molecular weight [MW], 3.472 kDa) is cleared from the blood by a combination of binding to natriuretic peptide receptors, enzymatic cleavage by neutral endopeptidases, and renal clearance. BNP is unstable in blood samples, because proteolytic enzymes continue to degrade BNP once blood is collected. For optimum recovery, BNP should be collected in plastic tubes containing EDTA as an anticoagulant, and testing should be conducted as soon after blood collection as possible [1]. Serum and heparinized plasma cannot be used for BNP testing. If samples cannot be tested within a few hours, they should be preserved by the addition of a protease inhibitor [2] or the centrifuged plasma can be stored frozen until analysis. Before inactivation by proteases, one investigator found that the two amino acids (serine-proline) from the N-terminal sequence are quickly lost [3]. Assays that have antibodies directed toward the N-terminal sequence (eg, Biosite) therefore may exhibit even less analyte stability than assays with antibodies directed toward the C-terminal sequence.

The metabolism of NT-proBNP (MW, 8.460 kDa) is not as well studied, partly because this protein does not have physiologic activity. The current interest relates to the usefulness of NT-proBNP as a biomarker for heart failure. Various techniques, including size-exclusion liquid chromatography, physicochemical techniques of analytical sedimentation, equilibrium ultracentrifugation, and circular dichroism, have demonstrated that NT-proBNP circulates in blood as

---

* Clinical Chemistry Laboratory, San Francisco General Hospital, 1001 Potrero Avenue, San Francisco, CA 94110.
E-mail address: wualan@labmed2.ucsf.edu

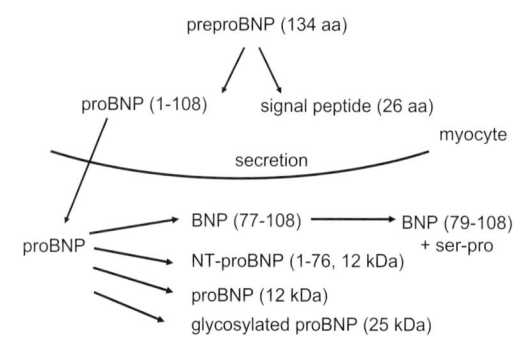

Fig. 1. Release of BNP and NT-proBNP from precursor forms in the heart.

a monomeric protein [4]. This recent report contradicts earlier studies that suggested that NT-proBNP exists in blood as a trimer [5]. In the absence of receptors, NT-proBNP is likely cleared by a combination of proteases and renal clearance. One investigator has shown that BNP is degraded from the N- and C-terminus ends of the protein [6]. Optimum detection of NT-proBNP is achieved by directing antibodies toward the central part of the molecule. Under these conditions, NT-proBNP is considerably more stable than BNP and can be stored for at least 72 hours at 4° C. Moreover, serum and heparinized plasma can be used in addition to EDTA blood collection tubes. These characteristics enable NT-proBNP to be more easily used than BNP for retrospective cardiac studies on blood previously collected and stored for other purposes.

Several studies have shown that the precursor protein, proBNP (MW, ~12 kDa), also circulated in blood of healthy patients and those who had heart failure [7]. Recently, Schellenberger and colleagues [8] demonstrated that plasma from patients with heart failure released a peptide that had a molecular weight of ~25 kDa. Treatment with deglycosylation enzymes produced the native BNP form. Further analysis revealed seven different sites of proBNP glycosylation. In summary, blood from heart failure patients contains BNP, NT-proBNP, proBNP, and glycosylated proBNP. The presence of these various forms must be considered when results of BNP and NT-proBNP assays are compared.

History of commercial diagnostic assays for natriuretic peptides

The patent for the use of BNP in heart failure is owned by Scios Inc. (Fremont, California), a biopharmaceutical company that manufacturers recombinant BNP (nesiritide) for therapeutic purposes. Scios was acquired by Johnson & Johnson (New Brunswick, New Jersey) in 2003. Before their acquisition, Scios sold licenses for BNP diagnostic products to Shionogi & Co., Ltd. (Osaka, Japan), Biosite Diagnostics (San Diego, California), and Abbott Laboratories (Abbott Park, Illinois). The first commercial immunoassay for BNP was developed during the 1990s by Shionogi. This radioimmunoassay is sold for "research use only" and has not been cleared by the FDA. The first FDA-cleared BNP assay was awarded to Biosite in November 2000. In 2003, Beckman Instruments acquired an agreement with Biosite to commercialize BNP on Beckman's automated immunoassay platforms (eg, Access 2) using Biosite antibodies and calibrators. There is therefore good but not total harmonization between the Biosite and Beckman assays. A cut-off concentration for BNP for heart failure diagnosis has been established at 100 pg/mL. Bayer Diagnostics (Tarrytown, New York) acquired a license from Shionogi & Co. and received FDA clearance for BNP on the Centaur and ACS:180 in 2003. Although Bayer uses the same antibodies from Shionogi, they have calibrated their assay such that a 100 pg/mL cut-off concentration can be used, and results are higher for Bayer analyzers than for the Shionogi assay. Response Biomedical Corp. (Burnaby, British Columbia, Canada) has also received a license from Shionogi for BNP. Abbott Laboratories through its manufacturing partner, Axis Shield, received FDA clearance in early 2004 for BNP on the AxSYM. The Tosoh Corp. (Tokyo, Japan) also has a BNP assay on their AIA series immunochemistry analyzers. Because of licensing restrictions, this assay is currently only available in Japan.

The patent for the use of NT-proBNP in heart failure is owned by Roche Diagnostics (Indianapolis, Indiana), who received FDA clearance for this assay in November 2002. Roche has subsequently licensed NT-proBNP to Dade Behring (Deerfield, Illinois), who received FDA clearance in December 2004, and to Inverness Medical, Response Biomedical (who have rights to both BNP, through Shionogi, and NT-proBNP, through bioMerieux [Marcy l'Etoile, France]), and bioMerieux. As part of the terms for the licensure, all NT-proBNP assays make use of the same antibody pairs and calibrators obtained from Roche. Results therefore are expected to be harmonized across platforms.

Current commercial BNP/NT-proBNP assays and cut-offs for heart failure

The use of BNP and NT-proBNP assays today in the United States can be estimated by subscriptions to the College of American Pathologists (CAP) Proficiency Survey. According to the 2006-A survey, there were 3408 laboratories who participated in this survey. Table 1 illustrates the breakdown of users according to manufacturers. For BNP, 50% of laboratories (1707 of 3408) reported using the Biosite Triage point-of-care meter. Although the CAP does not document where BNP testing is actually performed, most of these laboratories use the Triage meter within the central laboratory. The actual use of point-of-care testing (POCT) assays for BNP is expected to increase with the introduction of BNP on the iSTAT Analyzer (Abbott Diagnostics). The laboratories reporting NT-proBNP constitute 14% of the total for the sum of NT-proBNP and BNP (476 of 3408). The relative distribution of NT-proBNP users in Europe is higher than in the United States, although the total fraction of hospitals doing any natriuretic peptide testing is much lower than in the United States. Of the users of NT-proBNP, only 6.5% reported using a point-of-care instrument from the CAP survey (31 of 476). This will increase with the development and clearance of other point-of-care NT-proBNP assays. For comparative purposes, the total number of laboratories participating in BNP/NT-proBNP was higher than troponin (2653 for cTnI and 275 for cTnT), CK-MB mass assay (2399 total laboratories) and myoglobin (887 total laboratories) from the 2006 CAP Cardiac Marker-B survey. The use of these latter two markers has steadily declined over the past 5 years.

Table 1
Participants in the 2006 College of American Pathologists BNP-A survery

BNP Manufacturer	No. labs	NT-proBNP Manufacturer	No. labs
Abbott		Dade Behring	
AxSYM	248	Dimension	155
Architech	38	Stratus CS	31
Bayer		Roche	
ACS:180	34	E170	61
Centaur	445	Elecsys 1010/1020	229
Biosite Triage	1707		
Beckman Coulter	460		
Totals	2932		476

The cut-off concentration for use of BNP in the diagnosis of heart failure was established at 100 pg/mL by investigators of the Breathing Not Properly Trial using the Biosite Triage device [9]. For emergency department patients who present with acute dyspnea, this cut-off was optimized to increase the negative predictive value of the test and produced a clinical sensitivity and specificity for heart failure of 90% and 76%, respectively. To increase the positive predictive value of the test, some investigators have recommended use of a 500 pg/mL cut-off concentration [10]. BNP values between these limits are in a gray zone.

The cut-off concentration for NT-proBNP has been established by the manufacturer. For patients younger than 75 years of age, the cut-off is 125 pg/mL, and for patients aged 75 years or older, the cutoff is 450 pg/mL. In a study similar to the Breathing Not Properly Trial, the Pro-BNP Investigation of Dyspnea in the Emergency Department (PRIDE) study suggested cut-offs of 450 pg/mL for patients younger than age 50 years and 900 pg/mL for patients aged 50 years and older [11]. These cut-offs for NT-proBNP produced similar clinical performances to the BNP test observed in the BNP trial and are probably more appropriate than the manufacturer's recommendations.

Design and analytical correlation between commercial immunoassays

Fig. 2 shows the molecular structure and amino acid sequence of BNP and NT-proBNP. Although single-antibody competitive immunoassays have been developed for BNP, all commercial assays are currently two-site "sandwich" assays making use of a capture antibody to a bead or paramagnetic particle, and a detection antibody labeled to a radiotracer, fluorometric, or chemiluminescent tag. Table 2 lists the antibodies used in the various commercial BNP assays. All BNP assays have one antibody directed toward the ring structure and another at either the C-terminal sequences (Shionogi and Bayer) or the N-terminal sequence (Biosite and Beckman). The Roche NT-proBNP assay has antibodies that recognize the mid-molecule and the N-terminus. As shown in Fig. 2, the NT-proBNP fragment does not have a ring structure. Assay for BNP and NT-proBNP are expected to also recognize the prohormone, because the epitope sequences for proBNP are available for binding. The concentration of proBNP relative to BNP and NT-proBNP in healthy individuals and those who have heart

Enzymatic cleavage of pro-BNP

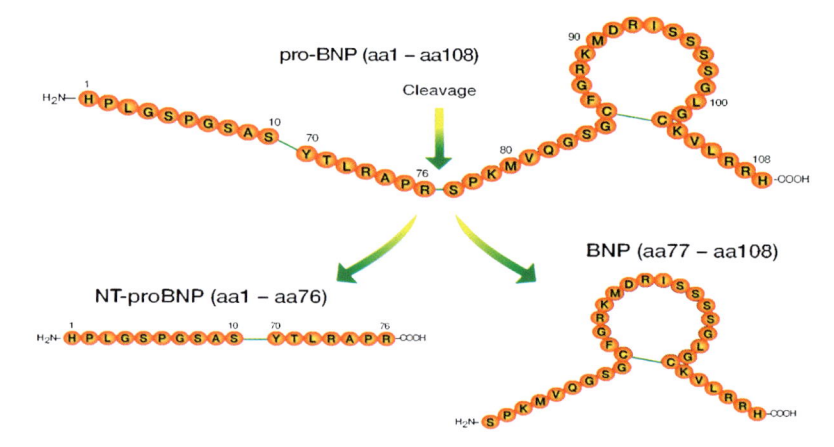

Fig. 2. Amino acid sequence of B-type natriuretic peptide and NT-proBNP. (*From* Omland T, Hall C. N-terminal pro-B-type natriuretic peptide. In: Wu AHB, editor. Cardiac markers. 2nd edition. Totowa (NJ): Humana Press; 2003; with permission.)

failure is currently unknown. Recently an assay has been developed that recognizes intact proBNP with no significant cross-reactivity toward the native hormone (BNP) or the inactive metabolite (NT-proBNP) [12]. Although the performance of this assay has not been tested in clinical studies, it is expected to be equal to that of BNP and NT-proBNP.

The analytical correlation between commercial BNP and NT-proBNP assay has been extensively studied in published reports and is summarized in Table 3 [13–21]. Certain conclusions can be rendered from these data. As expected, analytical assays that use the same antibody and calibrators have the highest degree of harmonization (eg, Access versus Triage, Centaur versus ShionoRIA, and Dimension versus Elecsys 1010) with regression coefficients exceeding 0.95. Within the limit of assay imprecision, results from these pairs of testing platforms are interchangeable. In contrast, there are significant differences in slope bias (−22% to 55%) and linear regression (r < 0.94) in the analytical correlation for BNP assays that use different antibodies and calibrators (particularly Centaur versus Triage, and AxSYM versus Centaur). Fortunately each of these assays is calibrated such that the cut-off concentration is fixed at 100 pg/mL for all commercial BNP platforms. Fig. 3 illustrates how this is accomplished. Panel A shows the correlation of two BNP assays against the ideal correlation, ie, a slope of 1.0 and a *y*-intercept of 0. Results for Assay 2 consistently produce higher values, and therefore a proportionally higher cut-off concentration is necessary to make the assays clinically concordant. Panel B shows that the results for Assay 2 have been adjusted such that the BNP cut-off concentration of 100 pg/mL intersects with the ideal correlation line. Under this condition, although results continue to differ from one another, there

Table 2
Commercial natriuretic peptide assay characteristics[a]

Assay	Antigen	Capture Ab	Detection Ab
Abbott AxSYM BNP	BNP a.a. 1-32	Scios (ring)	Shionogi (C-terminus)
Bayer Centaur BNP	BNP a.a. 1-32	Shionogi (C-terminus)	Shionogi (ring)
Biosite Triage (Beckman Access) BNP	BNP a.a. 1-32	Scios (ring)	Biosite (not characterized)
Shionogi BNP	BNP a.a. 1-32	Shionogi (C-terminus)	Shionogi (ring)
Roche Elecsys (Dade Dimension) NT-proBNP	NT-proBNP 1-76	Roche (N-terminus)	Roche (central)
Bio-Rad (not FDA-approved)	ProBNP 1-108	Hinge 76 region (between BNP and NT-proBNP)	BNP (unspecified region)

[a] *Adapted from* Fred S. Apple, PhD, personal communication, 2006.

Table 3
Analytical correlation between manufacturers of BNP and NT-proBNP assays

Assays	Regression equation	r	Reference
BNP vs. BNP			
Access 2 vs. Triage	0.96x − 6 pg/mL	0.95	[13]
Centaur vs. Triage	0.78x + 6 pg/mL	0.92	[14]
Centaur vs. ShionoRIA	1.11x − 1 pg/mL	0.98	[14]
AxSYM vs. Triage	1.13x − 6 pg/mL	0.94	[13]
AxSYM vs. Centaur	1.55x − 10 pg/mL	0.99	[15]
AxSYM vs. ShionoRIA	1.49x − 21 pg/mL	0.93	[16]
NT proBNP vs. NT-proBNP			
Dimension Rxl vs. Elecsys 2010	0.84x − 0.43 pg/mL	NA	[17]
BNP vs. NT-proBNP			
E170 NT-proBNP vs. Triage	8.9x − 225 pg/mL	0.80	[13]
1010 NT-proBNP vs. Triage	6.29 + 101 pg/mL	0.62	[18]
2010 NT-proBNP vs. Triage	4.95 + 7.5 pg/mL	0.57	[19]
2010 NT-proBNP vs. Shionogi	4.53x + 3.7 pg/mL	0.74	[19]
2010 NT-proBNP vs. AxSYM	7.23x + 2.53 pg/mL	0.69	[20]
2010 NT-proBNP vs. Centaur	15.34x + 2400 pg/mL	0.48	[21]

can be agreement of results with respect to those being either both below or both above the same cut-off concentration. Using this approach, Rawlins and colleagues examined the degree of concordance between different BNP assays on a group of patients with and without heart failure [13]. Of 197 specimens tested, the concordance between Access versus Triage, Centaur versus Triage, and AxSYM versus Triage BNP assays was very good at 95%, 93%, and 92%, respectively.

The analytical comparison between BNP and NT-proBNP is not as tight. As shown in Table 3, the linear regression coefficient between BNP and NT-proBNP assays ranges from 0.48 to 0.80. Although these correlations are statistically significant, the deviations are such that a slope and intercept correction factor cannot be applied to convert results of one analyte to an equivalent result for the other analyte. Furthermore, the degree of clinical concordance between NT-proBNP and the Triage BNP assay was reported in one study at 84% [12], lower than the 92%–95% concordance between BNP assays. Despite these analytical differences, the clinical usefulness of BNP versus NT-proBNP has been shown by many investigators to be roughly equivalent [22–24]. A hospital therefore would not gain any differential clinical information by offering both tests on the same patient. One investigator, however, concluded that BNP was more useful for severe heart failure and that NT-proBNP was more discerning for early left ventricular dysfunction [25]. Nevertheless, most clinical laboratories select between BNP and NT-proBNP based on the commercial laboratory immunoassay instrumentation available to them for other tests and not based on the preference of one analyte over the other.

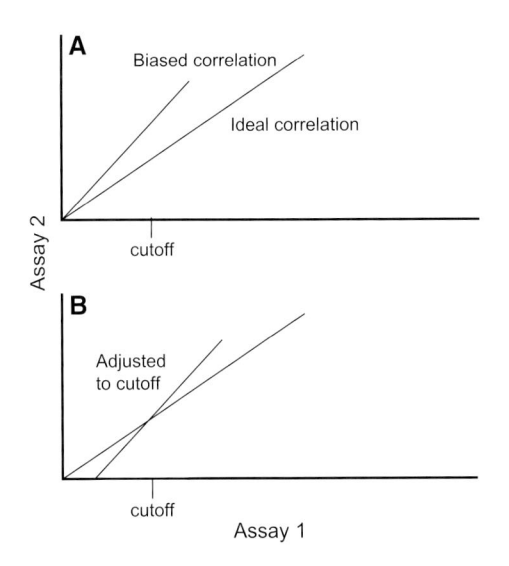

Fig. 3. (A) Comparison of two methods for BNP illustrating a proportional bias for results. Assay 2 has a proportional bias to Assay 1. (B) Adjustment of Assay 2 to harmonize the cutoff for Assay 1. Although results for Assay 2 continue to have a bias, both assays are within the limits of assay imprecision and should have concordance to each other with regard to samples that have either both normal or both abnormal concentrations. See text for details.

Cross-reactivities of BNP to other natriuretic-like peptides and substances

B-type natriuretic peptide constitutes a family of peptides with related chemical structures. As shown in Fig. 4, BNP is a 32-amino acid peptide with peptide hormone consisting of a ring structure of 17 amino acids, an N-terminus tail of 9 amino acids, and a C-terminus tail of 6 amino acids. Other natriuretic peptides that circulate in human blood include atrial natriuretic peptide (ANP), C-type natriuretic peptide (CNP), and urodilatin. Each of these peptides also contains a 17-member ring structure. There are 11 amino acids from this rink that are common to all members of the natriuretic peptide family. The other six members in the rink structure are unique. Moreover, the amino acids in the N- and C-terminus are different from each member of the natriuretic peptide family in number of residues and their amino acid identity.

For optimum analytical specificity, antibodies used in commercial BNP assays must be directed toward the amino sequences that are unique to BNP. This is particularly important for the antibody to the rink structure given this high degree of homology. For accurate analysis of BNP, manufacturers have conducted cross-reactivity studies for their assay and from package inserts, have reported no cross-reactivity toward the ANP family of peptides (ANP, preproANP, proANP, NT-proANP), CNP, urodilatin, NT-proBNP (for BNP assays), and BNP (for NT-proBNP assays). Other hormones should be tested that do not have structural homology to BNP but participate in volume and electrolyte balance, including aldosterone, angiotensin I, II, III, endothelin, adrenomedullin, and renin. Also drugs that are used in treating patients who have heart failure and acute coronary syndromes should be tested, including β-blockers, angiotensin converting enzyme inhibitors, angiotensin II antagonists, diuretics, heparin, nitrates, salicylates, clopidogrel, glycoprotein IIb/IIIa receptor inhibitors, and so on. None of the existing commercial assays report interferences with any of these compounds at concentrations exceeding expected physiologic, pathologic, or therapeutic levels.

Summary

The availability of two biomarkers for the same clinical indication, BNP and NT-proBNP for heart failure, has contributed to considerable confusion among cardiologists and clinicians. A similar situation has occurred over the last decade for cardiac troponins T and I. Given that the performance of these markers is similar, it would have been ideal to have a single marker for heart failure instead of two. Unfortunately issues regarding intellectual property rights have restricted availability of a manufacturer to license

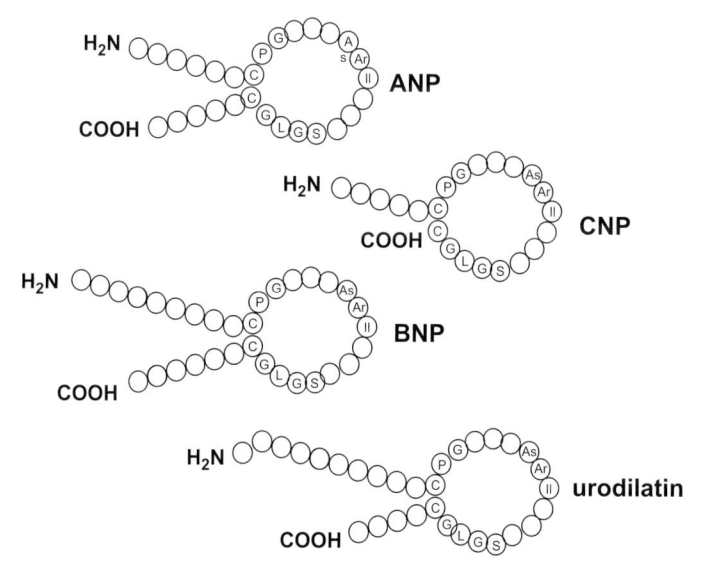

Fig. 4. Comparison of the amino acid structure of BNP versus ANP, CNP, and urodilatin. Amino acids that are labeled are conserved across these peptides and amino acids that are not labeled are different for the different peptides.

and make available only one marker at the expense of the other. Soon, a third marker, proBNP (Bio-Rad Laboratories) will be commercially available that has similar clinical performance to BNP and NT-proBNP and will add to the menu of available heart failure tests. Furthermore, there may also be other biomarkers available for heart failure that are not in the natriuretic peptide family, such as ST-2 [26]. Given that BNP and NT-proBNP are now well established, new biomarkers will have to offer additional diagnostic advantages that justify the expense of research and development, clinical trials, FDA clearance, and marketing of tests for these analytes. One area of active investigation is the discovery of protein and genetic biomarkers that can predict progression of asymptomatic patients who have hypertension and ischemic heart disease into overt heart failure [27]. These tests will have significant clinical impact if results can be linked to therapeutics that retard or prevent heart failure progression in a given patient.

References

[1] Shimizu H, Aono K, Masuta K, et al. Degradation of human brain natriuretic peptide (BNP) by contact activation of blood coagulation system. Clin Chim Acta 2001;305:181–6.

[2] Belenky A, Smith A, Zhang B, et al. The effect of class-specific protease inhibitors on the stabilization of B-type natriuretic peptide in human plasma. Clin Chim Acta 2004;340:163–72.

[3] Shimizu H, Masuta K, Aono K, et al. Molecular forms of human brain natriuretic peptide in plasma. Clin Chim Acta 2002;316:129–35.

[4] Crimmins DL. Human N-terminal proBNP is a monomer. Clin Chem 2005;51:1035–8.

[5] Seidler T, Pemberton C, Yandle T, et al. The amino terminal regions of proBNP and proANP oligomerise through leucine zipper-like coiled motifs. Biochem Biophys Res Commun 1999;255:495–501.

[6] Ala-Kopsala M, Magga J, Peuhkurinen K, et al. Molecular heterogeneity has a major impact on the measurement of circulating N-terminal fragments of A- and B-type natriuretic peptides. Clin Chem 2004;50:1576–88.

[7] Yandle TG, Richards AM, Gilbert A, et al. Assay of brain natriuretic peptide (BNP) in human plasma: evidence for high molecular weight BNP as a major plasma component in heart failure. J Clin Endocrinol Metab 1993;76:832–8.

[8] Schellenberger U, O'Rear J, Guzzetta A, et al. The precursor to B-type natriuretic peptide is an O-linked glycoprotein. Arch Biochem Biophys 2006;451:160–6.

[9] Maisel AS, Krishnaswamy P, Nowak RM, et al. Rapid measurement of B-type natriuretic peptide in the emergency diagnosis of heart failure. N Engl J Med 2002;347:161–7.

[10] Silver MA, Maisel A, Yancy CW. BNP Consensus Panel 2004: a clinical approach for the diagnostic, prognostic, screening, treatment monitoring, and therapeutic roles of natriuretic peptides in cardiovascular disease. Cong Heart Fail 2004;10(Suppl 3):1–30.

[11] Januzzi JL Jr, Camargo CA, Anwaruddin S, et al. The N-terminal Pro-BNP Investigation of Dyspnea in the Emergency Department (PRIDE) Study. Am J Cardiol 2005;95:948–54.

[12] Giuliani I, Rieunier F, Larue C, et al. Assay for measurement of intact B-type natriuretic peptide prohormone in blood. Clin Chem 2006;52:1054–61.

[13] Rawlins ML, Owen WE, Roberts WL. Performance characteristics of four automated natriuretic peptide assays. Am J Clin Pathol 2005;123:439–45.

[14] Wu AHB, Packer M, Smith A, et al. Analytical and clinical evaluation of the Bayer ADVIA Centaur automated B-type natriuretic peptide assay in patients with heart failure: a multisite study. Clin Chem 2004;50:867–73.

[15] Clerico A, Prontera C, Emdin M, et al. Analytical performance and diagnostic accuracy of immunometric assays for the measurement of plasma B-type natriuretic peptide (BNP) and N-terminal proBNP. Clin Chem 2005;51:445–7.

[16] Mueller T, Gegenhuber A, Poelz W, et al. Preliminary evaluation of the AxSYM B-type natriuretic peptide (BNP) assay and comparison with the ADVIA Centaur BNP assay. Clin Chem 2004;50:1104–6.

[17] Di Serio F, Ruggieri V, Varraso L, et al. Analytical evaluation of the Dade Behring Dimension RxL automated N-terminal proBNP (NT-proBNP) method and comparison with the Roche Elecsys 2010. Clin Chem Lab Med 2005;43:1263–73.

[18] Yeo KTJ, Wu AHB, Apple FS, et al. Multicenter evaluation of the Roche NT-proBNP assay and comparison to the Biosite Triage BNP assay. Clin Chim Acta 2003;338:107–15.

[19] Sokoll LJ, Baum H, Collinson PO, et al. Multicenter analytical performance evaluation of the Elecsys proBNP method. Clin Chem Lab Med 2004;42:965–73.

[20] Chien TI, Chen HH, Kao JT. Comparison of Abbott AxSYM and Roche Elecsys 2010 for measurement of BNP and NT-proBNP. Clin Chim Acta 2006;369:95–9.

[21] Sykes E, Karcher RE, Eisenstadt J, et al. Analytical relationship among Biosite, Bayer, and Roche methods for BNP and NT-proBNP. Am J Clin Pathol 2005;123:584–90.

[22] Yeo KT, Dumont KE, Brough T. Elecsys NT-proBNP and BNP assays: are there analytically and clinically relevant differences? J Card Fail 2005;11(5 Suppl):S84–8.

[23] Melanson SE, Lewandrowski EL. Laboratory testing for B-type natriuretic peptides (BNP and NT-proBNP): clinical usefulness, utilization, and impact on hospital operations. Am J Clin Pathol 2005; 124(Suppl):S122–8.

[24] Alibay Y, Beauchet A, El Mahmoud R, et al. Plasma N-terminal pro-brain natriuretic peptide and brain natriuretic peptide in assessment of acute dyspnea. Biomed Pharmacother 2005;59:20–4.

[25] Mueller T, Gegenhuber A, Poelz W, et al. Biochemical diagnosis of impaired left ventricular ejection fraction—comparison of the diagnostic accuracy of brain natriuretic peptide (BNP) and aminoterminal proBNP (NT-proBNP). Clin Chem Lab Med 2004; 42:159–63.

[26] Weinberg EO, Shimpo M, Hurwitz S, et al. Identification of serum soluble ST2 receptor as a novel heart failure biomarker. Circulation 2003;07: 721–6.

[27] Genome Canada. Protein expression profiling platforms for heart disease biomarker discovery. Available at: http://www.genomecanada.ca/xresearchers/researchPrograms/projects/projects.asp?1=e&id=s1p06. Accessed on May 17, 2006.

Natriuretic Peptides as Diagnostic Test: Lessons From the First 5 Years of Clinical Application

Lori B. Daniels, MD[a], Alan S. Maisel, MD[a,b,*]

[a]University of California San Diego, San Diego, CA, USA
[b]Veterans Affairs Medical Center, San Diego, CA, USA

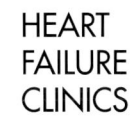

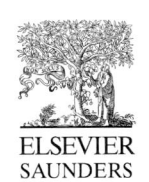

Heart failure can be a challenging diagnosis to make in the acute setting because of its many faces and nonspecific signs and symptoms. Because heart failure is not a single entity but a clinical syndrome resulting from many subordinate diseases, the clinical spectrum of patients who present with heart failure is broad. While practically and traditionally there is no substitute for a thorough history and physical examination, when dealing with acute heart failure diagnosis several recent studies have shown that these low-tech staples of our diagnostic armamentarium are often in need of reinforcement in the form of newer diagnostic tests. Measurement of natriuretic peptides is quickly becoming a go-to test that can help clinch the diagnosis in otherwise confusing cases.

Difficulty of diagnosing heart failure

Although textbooks teach us that patients with acute congestive heart failure (CHF) will present complaining of orthopnea, dyspnea, and paroxysmal nocturnal dyspnea, and that a careful examination will reveal their elevated jugular veins, lung rales, S3 heart sounds, and pitting peripheral edema, patients in real life rarely present as a textbook reads. It has been well documented that the signs and symptoms of heart failure are nonspecific and insensitive markers [1]. Chest radiography, electrocardiography, and standard laboratory assessments can sometimes help but do not always reveal classic findings. Echocardiography is currently the gold standard for diagnosing heart failure, but besides its limited availability, it can still leave room for confusion in a number of settings, including those patients with heart failure and normal systolic function.

Natriuretic peptides have emerged as a valuable tool for assisting with the diagnosis of heart failure. Readily available and relatively inexpensive, measurement of natriuretic peptides is now standard in many emergency departments (EDs) and clinics in evaluating patients with dyspnea and suspected heart failure.

B-type natriuretic peptide and the N-terminal fragment of pro B-type natriuretic peptide

B-type natriuretic peptide (BNP) and the amino-terminal fragment of pro-BNP (NT-proBNP) are secreted by the myocardium in response to increased end-diastolic wall stress. BNP, with a half-life of about 20 minutes, is quickly cleared via several mechanisms, including degradation and clearance by the natriuretic peptide receptor-C. In addition, BNP is degraded by neutral endopeptidase, and direct renal filtration and passive excretion may be responsible for some BNP clearance as well [2]. Despite 1:1 secretion of BNP and NT-proBNP, the longer half-life of NT-proBNP (about 1 to 2 hours) leads to higher circulating levels and slower fluctuations compared with BNP [3,4].

This work was supported by a grant from the American Heart Association (LBD).

* Corresponding author. Veterans Affairs Medical Center, Cardiology 111-A, 3350 La Jolla Village Drive, San Diego, CA 92161.
  E-mail address: amaisel@ucsd.edu (A.S. Maisel).

Major studies establishing the utility of natriuretic peptides for diagnosing acute congestive heart failure

Strong and consistent data establish the value of natriuretic peptides for facilitating the diagnosis of heart failure in patients presenting with dyspnea. Davis and colleagues [5] first measured levels of the natriuretic hormones atrial natriuretic peptide (ANP) and BNP in 52 patients presenting with acute dyspnea. They found that admission plasma BNP concentration more accurately reflected the final diagnosis than did left ventricular ejection fraction or ANP plasma concentration. Dao and colleagues [6] were the first to use the point-of-care BNP assay as they evaluated 250 patients presenting to an urgent care center with the chief complaint of dyspnea. Physicians assigned to the ED were asked to make an assessment of the probability (low, medium, or high) of heart failure for each dyspneic patient and were blinded to the results of BNP measurements. The finding that BNP levels were the strongest predictor of those who had heart failure spurred the international Breathing Not Properly study, the first large-scale prospective study using BNP levels to evaluate the cause of dyspnea.

Breathing Not Properly trial

The Breathing Not Properly trial prospectively evaluated 1586 patients who presented to the ED with acute dyspnea [7]. All patients received a standard workup as well as a bedside BNP measurement. Treating physicians were blinded to BNP levels and were asked to make an assessment of the probability of heart failure. The final diagnosis of heart failure was adjudicated by two cardiologists who, while blinded to BNP levels, had access to data such as subsequent echocardiography and the hospital course. BNP levels by themselves were found to be more accurate predictors of the presence or absence of heart failure than any historical or physical findings or laboratory values (Fig. 1). BNP levels were much higher in patients with subsequent heart failure than in patients with noncardiac dyspnea (675 pg/mL versus 110 pg/mL). A BNP cutoff value of 100 pg/mL had a sensitivity of 90% and a specificity of 76% for differentiating heart failure from other causes of dyspnea, and a cutoff level of 50 pg/mL had a negative predictive value of 96%. Pretest probability demonstrated a 43% indecision rate among physicians in the ED trying to make a diagnosis in patients with dyspnea. BNP levels added significantly to the tools of the clinician. Had BNP levels been available, the indecision rate would have been cut down to roughly only 11%. In multivariate analysis, BNP levels always contributed to the diagnosis, even after taking into account features of the history and physical exam.

B-type Natriuretic Peptide for Acute Shortness of breath EvaLuation

The BNP for Acute Shortness of breath EvaLuation (BASEL) study extended the value

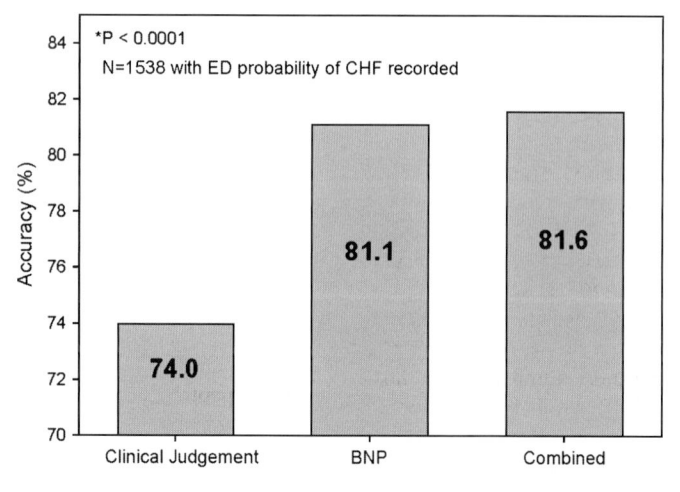

Fig. 1. Accuracy in the prediction of CHF using the emergency physician's clinical judgment alone, BNP > 100 pg/mL alone, or the combination of both. (*Adapted from* McCullough PA, Nowak RM, McCord J, et al. B-type natriuretic peptide and clinical judgement in emergency diagnosis of heart failure: Analysis from Breathing Not Properly (BNP) Multinational Study. Circulation 2002;106:420; with permission.)

ascertained from the Breathing Not Properly trial by demonstrating the cost-effectiveness of using BNP levels from the time of entry to the ED through the hospitalization phases of heart failure [8]. In the trial, the investigators studied patients presenting to the ED with acute dyspnea who were randomly assigned to undergo either a single measurement of BNP or no such measurement. Participating clinicians were advised that a level of BNP lower than 100 pg/mL made the diagnosis of heart failure unlikely, whereas a level higher than 500 pg/mL made it highly likely. For intermediate levels, use of clinical judgment and adjunctive testing were encouraged. In this single-blind trial of 452 patients, rapid measurement of BNP in the ED was associated with decreases in the rate of hospital admission by 10%, the median length of stay by 3 days, and the mean total cost of treatment by about $1800, with no adverse effects on mortality or the rate of subsequent hospitalization. This carefully performed trial suggests that the use of an inexpensive blood test for BNP in the emergency evaluation of acute dyspnea can significantly improve both the efficiency and the quality of care. These results are consistent with the Breathing Not Properly study and showed that the use of an improved diagnostic test in the ED can reduce the use of hospital resources and associated costs by eliminating the need for other, more expensive tests, or by establishing an alternative diagnosis that does not require hospitalization.

Rapid Emergency Department Heart Failure Outpatient Trial

The Rapid Emergency Department Heart Failure Outpatient Trial (REDHOT) study was designed to evaluate the relationship between BNP levels, clinical decision making in the ED, and clinical outcomes in heart failure patients [9]. It included 464 patients who presented to the ED with shortness of breath and who had BNP levels over 100 pg/mL. Treating physicians were blinded to BNP levels, and patients were followed for 90 days. Patients discharged from the ED had higher BNP levels than those admitted to the hospital. The median BNP level for discharged patients was 976 pg/mL, 27% higher than the median BNP level for patients who were admitted to the hospital (766 pg/mL). Yet BNP was the strongest predictor of ultimate 30- and 90-day outcomes. Approximately 90% of all patients were admitted to the hospital from the ED. Of the admitted patients, 11% had BNP levels lower than 200 pg/mL, which is indicative of less severe heart failure. Mortality for these patients was 0% at 30 days and only 2% at 90 days. Of the 10% of patients discharged from the ED, 78% had BNP levels above 400 pg/mL. At 30 days, mortality in these patients was 0%, but at 90 days, mortality was 9%. There was little mortality of those discharged with BNP levels under 400 pg/mL. Fig. 2 demonstrates the potential cost savings if low BNP levels could be used as a basis of ED discharge in 11% of all patients seen with CHF.

ProBNP Investigation of Dyspnea in the Emergency Department

Modeled after the Breathing Not Properly trial, the ProBNP Investigation of Dyspnea in the Emergency Department (PRIDE) study prospectively evaluated 600 patients presenting to the ED with acute dyspnea [10]. NT-proBNP levels were measured, and the results were compared with the clinical assessment of the managing physicians for identifying CHF. The authors suggested two different, age-based cut-points for diagnosing acute heart failure: NT-proBNP above 450 pg/mL for those younger than 50 years old, and NT-proBNP above 900 pg/mL for those 50 years or older. The study found that NT-proBNP was the strongest independent predictor of a final diagnosis of acute heart failure, with an odds ratio of 44. The optimal cut-point for ruling out heart failure was NT-proBNP less than 300 pg/mL, which had a 99% negative predictive value. This study helped establish the clinical utility of NT-proBNP for diagnosing or excluding CHF in the ED setting.

Comorbidities and special issues that influence the interpretation of B-type natriuretic peptide levels

While the Breathing Not Properly trial and the PRIDE study, among others, have helped to establish optimal cut-points for natriuretic peptides in diagnosing or excluding CHF, several caveats to these rules exist that can make natriuretic peptide levels seem discordant with the clinical picture.

Previous heart failure

Patients with a history of heart failure often have natriuretic peptide levels above the suggested cut-points, even when their volume status is

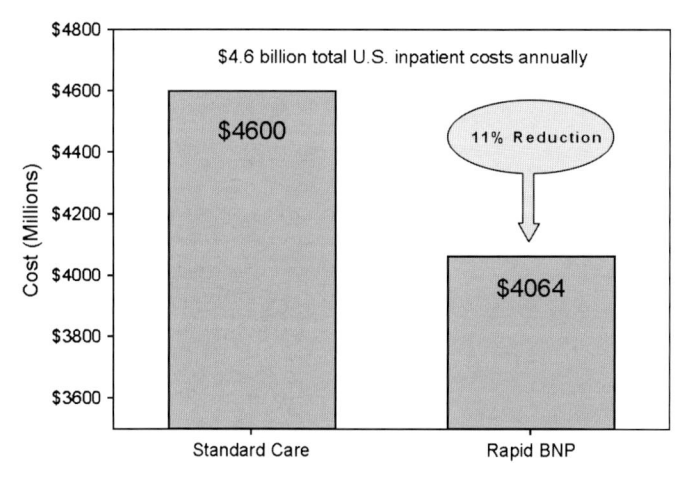

Fig. 2. Annual economic impact of BNP-guided emergency department discharge for patients with BNP less than 200 pg/mL. There is $506 million in annual savings for the "Rapid BNP"-guided strategy versus standard care. (*Data from* Maisel A, Hollander JE, Guss D, et al. Primary results of the Rapid Emergency Department Heart Failure Outpatient Trial (REDHOT): a multicenter study of B-type natriuretic peptide levels, emergency decision making, and outcomes in patients presenting with shortness of breath. J Am Coll Cardiol 2004;44(6):1328–33.)

optimal. This was demonstrated in the Breathing Not Properly trial, which showed that patients with a history of heart failure but without an acute exacerbation had intermediate levels of BNP in-between those without heart failure and those with an acute diagnosis of CHF [7]. For patients regularly followed in clinic, it may be beneficial to establish their "opti-volemic" or "dry weight" natriuretic peptide level, that is, the BNP or NT-proBNP level that corresponds to their optimized fluid status. Significant deviations above this value could then be used in lieu of traditional cut-points for diagnosing heart failure exacerbations, while values much lower than this opti-volemic level might indicate that the patient is over-diuresed or dry.

Advanced age

Both BNP and NT-proBNP levels increase with age [11–13]. Increased prevalence of heart disease with age, including diastolic dysfunction, may contribute to this phenomenon, but is probably not the principal factor. One study that excluded patients with "age-related" diastolic dysfunction, nonetheless found an association between age and elevated levels of BNP [14]. Other possible contributors include altered renal function, increased production, reduced secretion, or altered metabolism. Nevertheless, in the acutely dyspneic patient, the cut-point of 100 pg/mL for BNP was still found to be optimal [12].

Gender

Natriuretic peptide levels are higher in women than in men at any age [11,14]. Although the reason for the higher levels in women is unknown, estrogen may play a role, since a community-based study showed that older women on hormone replacement therapy had higher BNP levels than women not on therapy [14]. However, use of estrogen had only a minimal effect on NT-proBNP levels in the same cohort [13]. Again, these small differences are likely unimportant when dealing with the acutely dyspneic patient.

Pulmonary disease

It is often difficult to evaluate whether dyspnea is due to pulmonary disease or CHF. Although natriuretic peptide levels can be elevated in patients with pulmonary disease, levels are not usually elevated to the extent that they are in patients with heart failure. In a study of 321 patients with dyspnea who presented to the ED, BNP distinguished heart failure (mean BNP of 759 ± 798 pg/mL) from pulmonary disease (mean BNP 61 ± 10 pg/mL) and other clinical presentations with a high specificity and sensitivity [15]. The mean BNP values of patients with various pulmonary diseases are shown in Fig. 3. Moreover, when patients who had a history of heart failure but whose dyspnea was a result of chronic obstructive pulmonary disease (COPD)

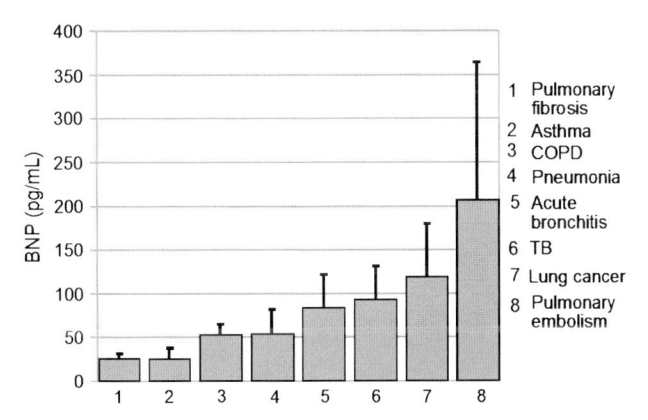

Fig. 3. Mean BNP values ± SD, in patients with various types of pulmonary disease. COPD, chronic obstructive pulmonary disease; TB, tuberculosis. (*Data from* Morrison LK, Harrison A, Krishnaswamy R, et al. Utility of a rapid B-natruiuretic peptide assay in differentiating congestive heart failure from lung disease in patients presenting with dyspnea. J Am Coll Cardiol 2002;39:207.)

(mean BNP 47 ± 23 pg/mL) were compared with patients who had a history of COPD but whose dyspnea was a result of heart failure (mean BNP 731 ± 764 pg/mL), a BNP value of 94 pg/mL yielded a sensitivity and specificity of 86% and 98%, respectively, and differentiated heart failure from lung disease with an accuracy of 91%.

Analysis of the results from the Breathing Not Properly multinational study found that using BNP could expose underlying CHF in patients with bronchospastic diseases such as asthma or COPD. Of 417 patients studied who had a history of asthma or COPD and no history of CHF, 87 (21%) were found to have a final diagnosis of CHF. The mean BNP levels for patients with and without a history of CHF were 587 pg/mL and 109 pg/mL, respectively. Therefore, routine natriuretic peptide testing in patients with a history of asthma or COPD increases the rate of new diagnosis of heart failure by 20% [16].

Acute respiratory distress syndrome

Acute respiratory distress syndrome (ARDS) is another potential cause of dyspnea in the emergency setting and can contribute to the difficulty in making accurate diagnoses in the ED. BNP levels were obtained from 35 patients with ARDS and 42 patients hospitalized with a diagnosis of heart failure [17]. The mean BNP value for those with ARDS was 123 pg/mL, significantly lower than the mean BNP value of 773 pg/mL for patients with CHF (Fig. 4). A cut-point of 360 pg/mL was determined to have a sensitivity of 90%, specificity of 86%, positive predictive value of 89%, and negative predictive value of 94% for differentiating between ARDS and CHF.

Pulmonary embolism

Acute, hemodynamically significant pulmonary embolism can cause elevation of natriuretic peptide levels. In this setting, natriuretic peptide levels are indicative of right heart strain rather than left heart failure. BNP still retains its prognostic value in this setting, as elevated levels portend worse outcomes in patients with pulmonary embolism [18]. It is important to remember in acutely dyspneic patients, that elevated natriuretic peptide levels are not pathognomonic for CHF, and acute pulmonary embolism must still be excluded, especially with "grey-zone" levels of BNP (100–500 pg/mL).

Lung disease with right heart failure

Similar to the scenario described for pulmonary emboli, the presence of severe lung disease with subsequent right heart dysfunction can cause elevated natriuretic peptide levels due to release of peptide from the right ventricular myocardium. This can be seen in chronic obstructive lung disease, primary pulmonary hypertension, and other causes of pulmonary hypertension [19–21]. Elevated BNP values in the setting of primary pulmonary hypertension have been shown to be strongly and independently associated with increased mortality rates [20].

Renal failure

Both BNP and NT-proBNP levels rise with worsening renal function, but it is unclear to what

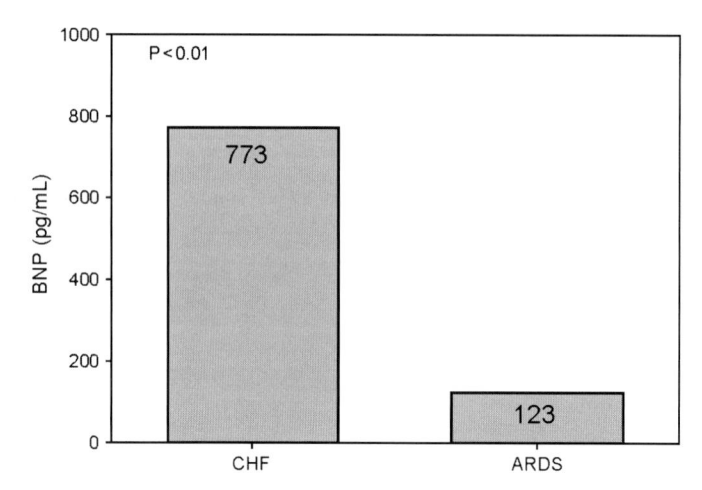

Fig. 4. BNP levels in CHF and ARDS. ARDS, acute respiratory distress syndrome. (*Data from* Berman B, Spragg R, Maisel A. B-type natriuretic peptide (BMP) levels in differentiating congestive heart failure from acute respiratory distress syndrome (ARDS). Abstracts from the 75th Annual Scientific Meeting of the American Heart Association. Circulation 2002;106(19):647.)

degree this rise is due to concomitant heart disease in patients with chronic kidney disease versus reduced clearance of natriuretic peptides from the circulation via renally mediated mechanisms. Several studies have found that BNP levels begin to rise at a threshold of estimated glomerular filtration rate (GFR) of 60 mL/min/1.7m^2, which is approximately the same level where increased rates of both systolic and diastolic heart failure are seen [22]. Regardless, an evaluation from the PRIDE study showed that NT-proBNP levels, although higher in patients with worse renal function, were still the strongest independent predictor of outcome in patients with GFR under 60 mL/min/1.7m^2 and suggested the higher cut-point of NT-proBNP above 1200 pg/mL for such patients [23]. Similarly, an analysis of the Breathing Not Properly trial also found a weak but significant correlation between GFR and BNP, and suggested a series of higher cut-points for those with GFR below 60 mL/min/1.7m^2 [24]. Recently, Vickery and colleagues [25] demonstrated a relatively larger increase in NT-proBNP versus BNP in patients with declining renal function (Table 1).

Acute coronary syndrome

Natriuretic peptide levels may rise in the setting of acute coronary syndrome, even without the presence of concomitant CHF. After myocardial infarction, BNP levels rise for about 24 hours, and then stabilize, with a second peak around day

Table 1
Patient characteristics by chronic kidney disease stage

	All stages	Stage 3	Stage 4	Stage 5	P
No. of patients	213	55	66	92	
GFR, mL/min/1.73 m^2	18.0	39.0	22.0	9.5	
Serum creatinine, mg/dL	3.3	1.7	2.9	5.7	<.0001
Plasma BNP, pg/mL	49.8	31.8	48.4	74.4	<.0001
Plasma NT-proBNP, pg/mL	753	279	575	1632	<.0001
NT-proBNP/BNP ratio	15.1	8.8	11.9	21.9	<.0001

Values expressed as median or number of patients.

Abbreviations: BNP, B-type natriuretic peptide; CKD, chronic kidney disease; GFR, glomerular filtration rate; NT-proBNP, N-terminal proBNP.

Adapted from Vickery S, Price CP, John RI, et al. B-type natriuretic peptide (BNP) and amino-terminal proBNP in patients with CKD: relationship to renal function and left ventricular hypertrophy. Am J Kidney Dis 2005;46:610–20.

5 to 8 [26,27]. The amount of rise may reflect the severity of left ventricular dysfunction [26]. Furthermore, an elevated BNP level in the setting of an acute coronary syndrome predicts the long-term risk of death or future cardiac events, independently of left ventricular function [28].

High-output states

Patients with high-output states including sepsis, cirrhosis, and hyperthyroidism can all present with elevated natriuretic peptide levels in the absence of overt heart failure. In patients with severe sepsis or septic shock, for example, natriuretic peptide levels may be markedly elevated [29,30]. The mechanisms responsible for this elevation are unknown, but may be related to BNP induction by endotoxin and other inflammatory mediators [31–33], or may reflect underlying myocardial dysfunction [34]. Similarly, patients with both alcoholic and nonalcoholic cirrhosis can have elevated natriuretic peptide levels that may reflect cardiac dysfunction or their hyperdynamic circulatory state [35–37]. Both BNP and NT-proBNP levels may be elevated in hyperthyroid patients compared with hypothyroid ones, and although levels may not exceed diagnostic cut-points, they do decrease with treatment of the hyperthyroid state [38,39]. Elevated BNP has also been reported in the setting of high-output cardiac failure caused by an oversized arteriovenous fistula in a hemodialysis patient [40].

Caveats: low levels of natriuretic peptides

Several scenarios can account for low levels of natriuretic peptides, even below diagnostic cut-points, despite the clear presence of heart failure. Keeping in mind the following caveats may help resolve clinical dilemmas that seem discrepant with natriuretic peptide values.

Obesity

Circulating levels of both BNP and NT-proBNP decrease with increasing body mass index, in patients both with and without heart failure [41–43]. Because of this, lower cut-points may be needed to reduce the false negative results for diagnosing heart failure in obese patients [44]. For patients with acute dyspnea and a body mass index of at least 35, a cut-point of BNP 54 pg/mL or higher maintains the same 90% sensitivity for diagnosing acute CHF as does the standard cut-point of BNP 100 pg/mL or higher in nonobese individuals (Fig. 5).

The pathophysiologic basis for lower natriuretic peptide levels in obesity remains debated. Although there is some evidence that natriuretic peptide receptors in adipose cells lead to increased clearance of BNP, there may also be a component of reduced natriuretic peptide secretion in obesity that helps account for the lower levels of NT-proBNP that are also seen. Despite the lower circulating levels, natriuretic peptides appear to retain their prognostic capacity in obese patients [45].

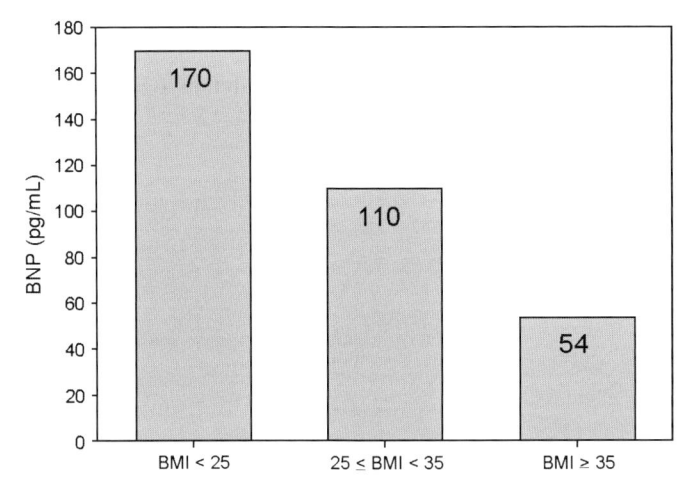

Fig. 5. BNP cut-point needed to maintain 90% sensitivity in diagnosing acute heart failure, based on BMI. Specificity at the 90% sensitivity level shown was at least 70% for all groups. BMI, body mass index. (*Adapted from* Daniels LB, Clopton P, Bhalla V, et al. How obesity affects the cut-points for B-type natriuretic peptide in the diagnosis of acute heart failure. Results from the Breathing Not Properly Multinational Study. Am Heart J 2006;151:1003; with permission.)

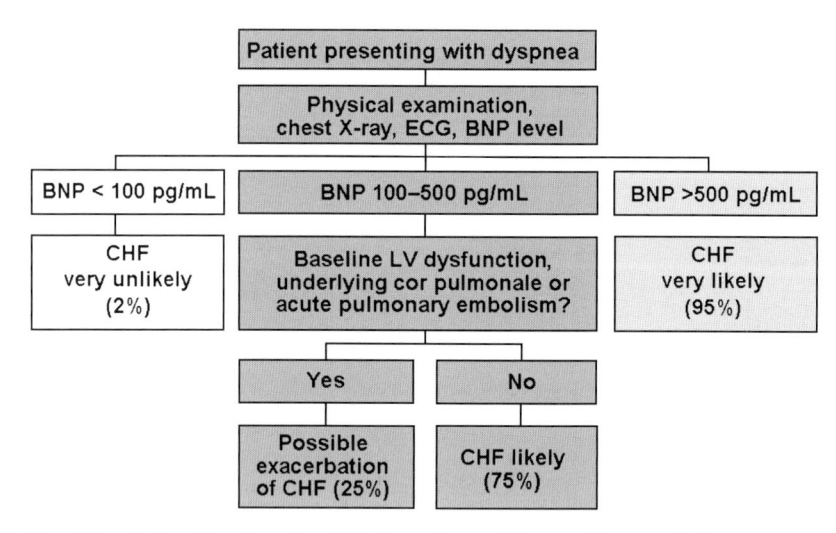

[Flowchart: Patient presenting with dyspnea → Physical examination, chest X-ray, ECG, BNP level. BNP < 100 pg/mL: CHF very unlikely (2%). BNP 100–500 pg/mL: Baseline LV dysfunction, underlying cor pulmonale or acute pulmonary embolism? Yes → Possible exacerbation of CHF (25%); No → CHF likely (75%). BNP >500 pg/mL: CHF very likely (95%).]

Fig. 6. Clinically validated algorithm for using BNP in patients with acute dyspnea. CHF, congestive heart failure; ECG, electrocardiogram; LV, left ventricular. (*Data from* Maisel AS, McCullough PA. Cardiac natriuretic peptides: a proteomic window to cardiac function and clinical management. Rev Cardiovasc Med 2003;4(Suppl 4):S7.)

Flash pulmonary edema

In patients presenting with a very rapid onset of heart failure symptoms of 1 hour or less, natriuretic peptide levels may seem inappropriately low. This is likely a result of the time required for natriuretic peptide up-regulation and expression in response to ventricular wall stress. BNP, unlike ANP, has only minimal storage in secretory granules; rather, it is primarily synthesized and secreted in bursts [46]. When a patient presents early in the setting of flash pulmonary edema, there may be insufficient time for gene expression to take place between the initial trigger (ie, wall stretch) and subsequent measurement of natriuretic peptide levels.

Congestive heart failure due to causes upstream from the left ventricle

When CHF is a result of causes upstream from the left ventricle, such as acute mitral regurgitation

"Rule in"

Age strata	Optimal cut-point	Sensitivity	Specificity	PPV	NPV	Accuracy
All <50 years (n=184)	450 pg/ml	97%	93%	76%	99%	95%
All 50-75 years (n=537)	900 pg/ml	90%	82%	83%	88%	85%
All >75 years (n=535)	1800 pg/ml	85%	73%	92%	55%	83%
Overall average		90%	84%	88%	66%	85%

"Rule out"

	Optimal cut-point	Sensitivity	Specificity	PPV	NPV	Accuracy
All patients (n=1256)	300 pg/ml	99%	60%	77%	98%	83%

Fig. 7. Clinically validated cut-points for NT-proBNP in patients with acute dyspnea. NPV, negative predictive value; PPV, positive predictive value. (*Data from* Januzzi JL, van Kimmenade R, Lainchbury J, et al. NT-proBNP testing for diagnosis and short-term prognosis in acute destabilized heart failure: an international pooled analysis of 1256 patients: the International Collaborative of NT-proBNP study. Eur Heart J 2006;27:335.)

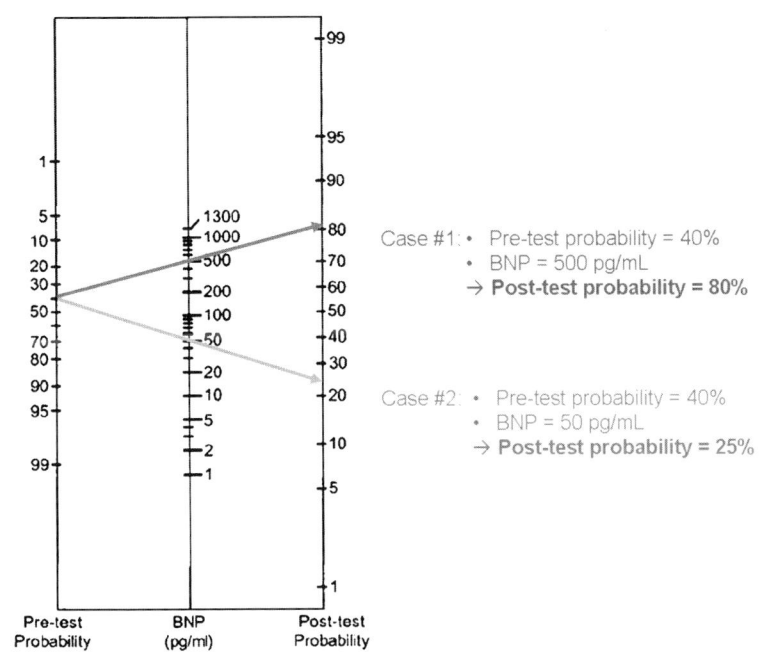

Fig. 8. Effect of various BNP levels in determining posttest probability of CHF for a given pretest probability. BNP aids in the diagnosis of acute heart failure in the setting of intermediate pretest probability. (*Adapted from* McCullough PA, Nowak RM, McCord J, et al. B-type natriuretic peptide and clinical judgment in emergency diagnosis of heart failure: analysis from Breathing Not Properly (BNP) Multinational study. Circulation 2002;106:420; with permission.)

or mitral stenosis, natriuretic peptide levels can be low or normal despite severe CHF. This is because left ventricular function may not be compromised in these patients, especially in the acute setting. Similarly, patients with constrictive pericarditis may have symptoms of heart failure and elevated filling pressures, but tend to have low natriuretic peptide levels due to lack of ventricular stretch [47].

Diagnostic algorithms

Figs. 6 and 7 show diagnostic algorithms for using BNP and NT-proBNP in the dyspneic patient. It should be noted that along with a natriuretic peptide level, a history, physical examination, chest x-ray, and electrocardiogram should be undertaken. For BNP, levels less than 100 pg/mL usually rule out CHF, while levels above 500 pg/mL usually rule in CHF. Interpretation of levels falling within the "grey-zone" (100–500 pg/mL) requires clinical expertise. For NT-proBNP there is a rule-out level less than 300 pg/mL and a rule-in level that is strongly based on age (Fig. 7).

Summary

Great strides have been made with regard to the importance of natriuretic peptide levels in the diagnosis of CHF in the acutely dyspneic patient. Not since the advent of echocardiography some 20 years ago have we had such an advance in making the appropriate and timely diagnosis of CHF. Fig. 8 shows perhaps the true value of natriuretic peptide values in this regard. Given an intermediate pretest probability based on history, physical exam, chest x-ray, and electrocardiogram, natriuretic peptide levels can substantially change our posttest probability of CHF. This can only lead to better outcomes for our patients.

References

[1] Stevenson LW, Perloff JK. The limited reliability of physical signs for estimating hemodynamics in chronic heart failure. JAMA 1989;261(6):884–8.
[2] Davidson NC, Struthers AD. Brain natriuretic peptide. J Hypertens 1994;12(4):329–36.
[3] Ruskoaho H. Cardiac hormones as diagnostic tools in heart failure. Endocr Rev 2003;24(3):341–56.

[4] McCullough PA, Sandberg KR. Sorting out the evidence on natriuretic peptides. Rev Cardiovasc Med 2003;4(Suppl 4):S13–9.

[5] Davis M, Espiner E, Richards G, et al. Plasma brain natriuretic peptide in assessment of acute dyspnoea. Lancet 1994;343(8895):440–4.

[6] Dao Q, Krishnaswamy P, Kazanegra R, et al. Utility of B-type natriuretic peptide in the diagnosis of congestive heart failure in an urgent-care setting. J Am Coll Cardiol 2001;37(2):379–85.

[7] Maisel AS, Krishnaswamy P, Nowak RM, et al. Rapid measurement of B-type natriuretic peptide in the emergency diagnosis of heart failure. N Engl J Med 2002;347(3):161–7.

[8] Mueller C, Scholer A, Laule-Kilian K, et al. Use of B-type natriuretic peptide in the evaluation and management of acute dyspnea. N Engl J Med 2004; 350(7):647–54.

[9] Maisel A, Hollander JE, Guss D, et al. Primary results of the Rapid Emergency Department Heart Failure Outpatient Trial (REDHOT). A multicenter study of B-type natriuretic peptide levels, emergency department decision making, and outcomes in patients presenting with shortness of breath. J Am Coll Cardiol 2004;44(6):1328–33.

[10] Januzzi JL Jr, Camargo CA, Anwaruddin S, et al. The N-terminal Pro-BNP investigation of dyspnea in the emergency department (PRIDE) study. Am J Cardiol 2005;95(8):948–54.

[11] Wang TJ, Larson MG, Levy D, et al. Impact of age and sex on plasma natriuretic peptide levels in healthy adults. Am J Cardiol 2002;90(3):254–8.

[12] Maisel AS, Clopton P, Krishnaswamy P, et al. Impact of age, race, and sex on the ability of B-type natriuretic peptide to aid in the emergency diagnosis of heart failure: results from the Breathing Not Properly (BNP) multinational study. Am Heart J 2004; 147(6):1078–84.

[13] Costello-Boerrigter LC, Boerrigter G, Redfield MM, et al. Amino-terminal pro-B-type natriuretic peptide and B-type natriuretic peptide in the general community: determinants and detection of left ventricular dysfunction. J Am Coll Cardiol 2006;47(2): 345–53.

[14] Redfield MM, Rodeheffer RJ, Jacobsen SJ, et al. Plasma brain natriuretic peptide concentration: impact of age and gender. J Am Coll Cardiol 2002; 40(5):976–82.

[15] Morrison LK, Harrison A, Krishnaswamy P, et al. Utility of a rapid B-natriuretic peptide assay in differentiating congestive heart failure from lung disease in patients presenting with dyspnea. J Am Coll Cardiol 2002;39(2):202–9.

[16] McCullough PA, Hollander JE, Nowak RM, et al. Uncovering heart failure in patients with a history of pulmonary disease: rationale for the early use of B-type natriuretic peptide in the emergency department. Acad Emerg Med 2003;10(3):198–204.

[17] Berman B, Spragg R, Maisel A. B-type natriuretic peptide (BNP) levels in differentiating congestive heart failure from acute respiratory distress syndrome (ARDS). Abstracts from the 75th Annual Scientific Meeting of the American Heart Association. Circulation 2002;106(19): SII-647.

[18] Kucher N, Printzen G, Goldhaber SZ. Prognostic role of brain natriuretic peptide in acute pulmonary embolism. Circulation 2003;107(20):2545–7.

[19] Bando M, Ishii Y, Sugiyama Y, et al. Elevated plasma brain natriuretic peptide levels in chronic respiratory failure with cor pulmonale. Respir Med 1999;93(7):507–14.

[20] Nagaya N, Nishikimi T, Uematsu M, et al. Plasma brain natriuretic peptide as a prognostic indicator in patients with primary pulmonary hypertension. Circulation 2000;102(8):865–70.

[21] Nagaya N, Nishikimi T, Okano Y, et al. Plasma brain natriuretic peptide levels increase in proportion to the extent of right ventricular dysfunction in pulmonary hypertension. J Am Coll Cardiol 1998;31(1):202–8.

[22] McCullough PA, Sandberg KR. B-type natriuretic peptide and renal disease. Heart Fail Rev 2003; 8(4):355–8.

[23] Anwaruddin S, Lloyd-Jones DM, Baggish A, et al. Renal function, congestive heart failure, and amino-terminal pro-brain natriuretic peptide measurement: results from the ProBNP Investigation of Dyspnea in the Emergency Department (PRIDE) Study. J Am Coll Cardiol 2006;47(1):91–7.

[24] McCullough PA, Duc P, Omland T, et al. B-type natriuretic peptide and renal function in the diagnosis of heart failure: an analysis from the Breathing Not Properly Multinational Study. Am J Kidney Dis 2003;41(3):571–9.

[25] Vickery S, Price CP, John RI, et al. B-type natriuretic peptide (BNP) and amino-terminal proBNP in patients with CKD: relationship to renal function and left ventricular hypertrophy. Am J Kidney Dis 2005;46(4):610–20.

[26] Morita E, Yasue H, Yoshimura M, et al. Increased plasma levels of brain natriuretic peptide in patients with acute myocardial infarction. Circulation 1993; 88(1):82–91.

[27] Talwar S, Squire IB, Downie PF, et al. Profile of plasma N-terminal proBNP following acute myocardial infarction: correlation with left ventricular systolic dysfunction. Eur Heart J 2000;21(18):1514–21.

[28] de Lemos JA, Morrow DA, Bentley JH, et al. The prognostic value of B-type natriuretic peptide in patients with acute coronary syndromes. N Engl J Med 2001;345(14):1014–21.

[29] Rudiger A, Gasser S, Fischler M, et al. Comparable increase of B-type natriuretic peptide and amino-terminal pro-B-type natriuretic peptide levels in patients with severe sepsis, septic shock, and acute heart failure. Crit Care Med 2006;34(8):2140–4.

[30] Jones AE, Kline JA. Elevated brain natriuretic peptide in septic patients without heart failure. Ann Emerg Med 2003;42(5):714–5.

[31] Tomaru Ki K, Arai M, Yokoyama T, et al. Transcriptional activation of the BNP gene by lipopolysaccharide is mediated through GATA elements in neonatal rat cardiac myocytes. J Mol Cell Cardiol 2002;34(6):649–59.

[32] Tanaka T, Kanda T, Takahashi T, et al. Interleukin-6-induced reciprocal expression of SERCA and natriuretic peptides mRNA in cultured rat ventricular myocytes. J Int Med Res 2004;32(1):57–61.

[33] Ma KK, Ogawa T, de Bold AJ. Selective upregulation of cardiac brain natriuretic peptide at the transcriptional and translational levels by pro-inflammatory cytokines and by conditioned medium derived from mixed lymphocyte reactions via p38 MAP kinase. J Mol Cell Cardiol 2004;36(4):505–13.

[34] Charpentier J, Luyt CE, Fulla Y, et al. Brain natriuretic peptide: a marker of myocardial dysfunction and prognosis during severe sepsis. Crit Care Med 2004;32(3):660–5.

[35] Yildiz R, Yildirim B, Karincaoglu M, et al. Brain natriuretic peptide and severity of disease in non-alcoholic cirrhotic patients. J Gastroenterol Hepatol 2005;20(7):1115–20.

[36] Wong F, Siu S, Liu P, et al. Brain natriuretic peptide: is it a predictor of cardiomyopathy in cirrhosis? Clin Sci (Lond) 2001;101(6):621–8.

[37] Henriksen JH, Gotze JP, Fuglsang S, et al. Increased circulating pro-brain natriuretic peptide (proBNP) and brain natriuretic peptide (BNP) in patients with cirrhosis: relation to cardiovascular dysfunction and severity of disease. Gut 2003;52(10):1511–7.

[38] Kohno M, Horio T, Yasunari K, et al. Stimulation of brain natriuretic peptide release from the heart by thyroid hormone. Metabolism 1993;42(8):1059–64.

[39] Schultz M, Faber J, Kistorp C, et al. N-terminal-pro-B-type natriuretic peptide (NT-pro-BNP) in different thyroid function states. Clin Endocrinol (Oxf) 2004;60(1):54–9.

[40] Jin H, Afonso L, Singh A, et al. Case report: recurrent heart failure with preserved ejection fraction but markedly elevated BNP in a 51-year-old female on hemodialysis with oversized AV fistula. Int J Cardiol 2006;110(3):429–30.

[41] Wang TJ, Larson MG, Levy D, et al. Impact of obesity on plasma natriuretic peptide levels. Circulation 2004;109(5):594–600.

[42] Mehra MR, Uber PA, Park MH, et al. Obesity and suppressed B-type natriuretic peptide levels in heart failure. J Am Coll Cardiol 2004;43(9):1590–5.

[43] Krauser DG, Lloyd-Jones DM, Chae CU, et al. Effect of body mass index on natriuretic peptide levels in patients with acute congestive heart failure: a ProBNP Investigation of Dyspnea in the Emergency Department (PRIDE) substudy. Am Heart J 2005;149(4):744–50.

[44] Daniels LB, Clopton P, Bhalla V, et al. How obesity affects the cut-points for B-type natriuretic peptide in the diagnosis of acute heart failure. Results from the Breathing Not Properly Multinational Study. Am Heart J 2006;151(5):1006–12.

[45] Horwich TB, Hamilton MA, Fonarow GC. B-type natriuretic peptide levels in obese patients with advanced heart failure. J Am Coll Cardiol 2006;47(1):85–90.

[46] Yoshimura M, Yasue H, Okumura K, et al. Different secretion patterns of atrial natriuretic peptide and brain natriuretic peptide in patients with congestive heart failure. Circulation 1993;87(2):464–9.

[47] Leya FS, Arab D, Joyal D, et al. The efficacy of brain natriuretic peptide levels in differentiating constrictive pericarditis from restrictive cardiomyopathy. J Am Coll Cardiol 2005;45(11):1900–2.

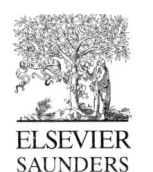

Diagnostic Applications of Natriuretic Peptides in Ischemic Heart Disease

Bertil Lindahl, MD, PhD*, Stefan James, MD, PhD

University Hospital of Uppsala, Uppsala, Sweden

Early assessment of patients who have symptoms suggestive of an acute coronary syndrome (ACS) remains a challenge considering the heterogeneity of underlying pathologies and clinical outcomes. The purpose of the early evaluation of these patients is threefold: first, to diagnose or exclude acute myocardial infarction (AMI) second, to identify patients at different risks for future cardiac events; and third, to be able to select appropriate treatment. Currently the initial assessment of these patients is based on the patient's history, clinical findings, ECG data, and serial testing of biochemical markers of myocardial necrosis, preferably troponin T or I. In the last few years, an increasing number of studies have evaluated the addition of the natriuretic peptides, NT-proBNP and BNP, in the diagnostic and prognostic arsenal for assessment of patients who have a suspected ACS. The studies of the value of natriuretic peptides have also been extended to patients who have stable angina pectoris for detection of significant coronary artery disease (CAD) and for assessment of the long-term risk.

NT-proBNP and BNP in the different forms of ischemic heart disease

The prognostic value of NT-proBNP and BNP has been evaluated in the full spectrum of ischemic heart disease in a large number of studies. It is striking that the increased mortality associated with elevation of NT-proBNP or BNP is of a similar degree, regardless of type of presentation of the ischemic heart disease.

Stable angina

Patients who have stable angina pectoris as a group have a low risk for cardiac events. The group is heterogeneous, however, and therefore identification of subgroups at different risk levels is justified. Several studies summarized in Table 1 have demonstrated the value of determination of NT-proBNP or BNP for this purpose [1–7]. In the study of Kragelund and colleagues [1], 1034 patients who had stable angina and were referred for coronary angiography were followed for a median of 9 years. The mortality increased by increasing quartiles of NT-proBNP and the survival curves continued to separate during the whole follow-up period (Fig. 1). The strong prognostic value remained also after adjustment for other known prognostic variables, including left ventricular ejection fraction (LVEF). Although the NT-proBNP level was significantly (negatively) associated with the LVEF ($P < .001$), the hazard ratio for death was essentially similar among patients who had LVEF greater than 60% and presence of significant CAD on angiography (HR, 1.9; 95% CI, 1.2–3.3) as the total study population (HR, 2.4; 95% CI, 1.5–4.0). That NT-proBNP and BNP are independent predictors of mortality also among patients who have normal systolic LVEF is verified in other studies [2,4–7].

Studies have also shown that elevation of NT-proBNP/BNP is associated with significant CAD on angiography independently of the LVEF [8,9].

Bertil Lindahl has received consulting fees, lecture fees, or grant support from Roche Diagnostics, Dade-Behring, Beckman Coulter, and Radiometer A/S.

* Corresponding author. Department of Cardiology and Uppsala Research Center, University Hospital of Uppsala, Uppsala SE 751-85, Sweden.
 E-mail address: bertil.lindahl@akademiska.se (B. Lindahl).

Table 1
Association between outcome and NT-proBNP/BNP levels in stable angina

Study	Endpoint	N	Marker	F-U	Cut-off	Adjusted OR or HR	(95% CI)
[1]	Death	1034	NT-proBNP	9 y	Quartiles	4th vs. 1st	2.4 (1.5–4.0)
[2]	Death	1059	NT-proBNP	3.6 y	Quartiles	4th vs. 1st	5.8 (2.1–16.4)
[3]	Death/MI	225	NT-proBNP	2.6 y	Quartiles	4th vs. 1st	3.7 (1.4–9.7)
[4]	CV death/MI	570	NT-proBNP	2.0 y	Quartiles	4th vs. 1st	4.0 (1.1–13.9)
[5]	Death/CHF	1049	NT-proBNP BNP	12 m	Median	—	2.1 (1.1–3.9) 1.9 (1.02–3.5)
[6]	Death	186	BNP	7.4 y	—	Per 10 ng/L increase	1.1 (1.03–1.2)
[7]	CV death/MI	1085	BNP	2.5 y	Quartiles	4th vs. 1st	6.1 (2.0–18.6)

Abbreviations: CI, confidence interval; F-U, follow-up time; HR, hazard ratio; N, number of patients; OR, odds ratio.

The ability to detect significant CAD is only modest, however, making NT-proBNP/BNP not clinically useful for diagnosis of significant CAD [8]. Whether measurement of NT-proBNP/BNP is useful for identification of patients who benefit from a particular treatment is unknown and future research should focus on this important issue.

Non–ST-elevation acute coronary syndromes

Patients who have non–ST-elevation acute coronary syndromes (non–STE-ACS) constitute a heterogeneous population with regard to their clinical history and the underlying cause of their symptoms. Consequently the prognosis is also subject to considerable variation. Early risk prediction is essential for the identification of patients at high risk and for the selection of the most appropriate treatment strategy. Moreover, with early risk-prediction, patients at low risk can be identified, and costly and potentially hazardous treatments and prolonged hospital stays can be avoided.

Several key studies of the prognostic value of NT-proBNP and BNP are summarized in Table 2 [10–15]. The first published study was by de Lemos and colleagues [10]. BNP was measured in a cohort including 2525 patients who had ACS, of which 1698 patients had unstable angina or non–ST-elevation AMI. In the group that had non–STE-ACS, the 10-month mortality increased with increasing levels of BNP, with a mortality of approximately 1% in the lowest quartile and 7% to 15% in the highest quartile. The same research group validated these findings in another study, showing again increasing mortality by increasing

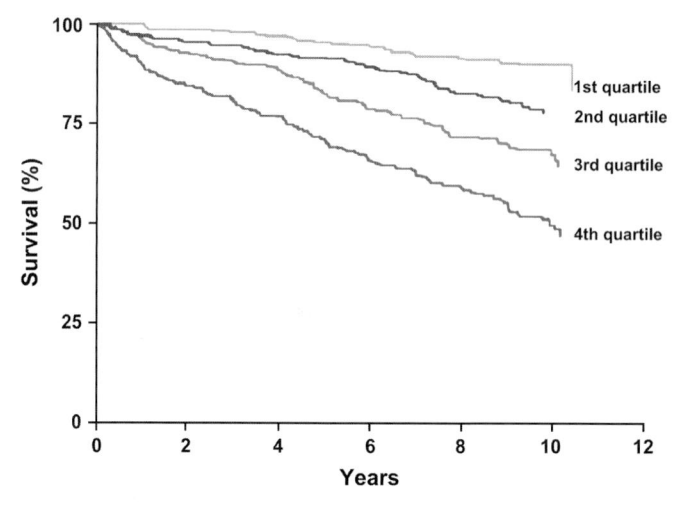

Fig. 1. Overall survival among patients who have stable CAD, according to quartiles of NT-proBNP. (*From* Kragelund C, Gronning B, Kober L, et al. N-terminal pro-B-type natriuretic peptide and long-term mortality in stable coronary heart disease. N Engl J Med 2005;352(7):672; with permission.)

Table 2
Association between outcome and NT-proBNP/BNP levels in non–ST-elevation ACS

Study	Endpoint	N	Marker	F-U	Cut-off	Adjusted OR or HR (95% CI)	
[10]	Death	2525[a]	BNP	10 m	Quartiles	4th vs. 1st	5.8 (1.7–19.7)
[11]	Death	1059	BNP	6 m	80 ng/L		3.3 (1.7–6.3)
[12]	Death/MI	775	NT-proBNP	35 m	Quartiles	4th vs. 1st	5.4 (2.0–14.4)
[13]	CV death/MI	504 non-STE-ACS	NT-proBNP	51 m	545 ng/L	Non–STEMI	2.3 (0.8–6.6)
						UA	2.0 (0.6–6.7)
[14]	Death	6609	NT-proBNP	12 m	669 ng/L		2.0 (1.5–2.6)
[15]	CV death	2019	NT-proBNP	24 m	Tertiles	Noninvasive[b]	3.8 (2.0–7.3)
						Invasive[c]	3.1 (1.5–6.5)

Abbreviations: CI, confidence interval; F-U, follow-up time; HR, hazard ratio; N, number of patients; Non–STEMI, non–ST-elevation myocardial infarction; OR, odds ratio; UA, unstable angina.
[a] 1698 with non–STE-ACS.
[b] 3rd vs. 1–2nd tertile in those randomized to a noninvasive treatment strategy.
[c] 3rd vs. 1–2nd tertile in those randomized to an invasive treatment strategy.

levels of BNP (Fig. 2) [11]. The prospectively defined decision-limit of 80 ng/L was able to identify a group of patients who had a 30-day and 6-month mortality of 5.0% and 8.4%, respectively, compared with 1.2% and 1.8% in the group that had lower levels of BNP. Similar to the first study, the level of BNP was strongly associated with mortality even when adjusted for well-known risk factors, such as age, gender, diabetes, ST-segment depression, history of congestive heart failure, heart failure at presentation, and baseline level of troponin. BNP was also associated with the risk for subsequent heart failure, whereas there was no significant association with the risk for future myocardial infarction (MI).

There are several studies evaluating NT-proBNP in patients who have non–STE-ACS. In the first study by the authors' group [12], NT-proBNP was analyzed on admission in a group of 755 patients consecutively admitted to coronary care unit because of symptoms suggestive of an ACS and no ST-segment elevations (407 with a final

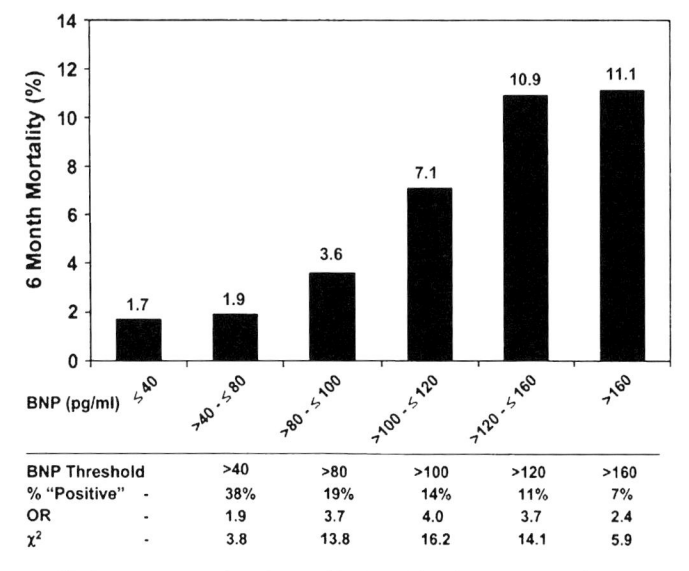

Fig. 2. Mortality risk stratified by B-type natriuretic peptide (BNP) levels over range of 40 to 160 pg/mL. The odds ratio (ORs) and chi-squared (χ^2) statistics in the table below the chart are based on BNP results dichotomized at the lower bound of the range. (*From* Morrow DA, de Lemos JA, Sabatine MS, et al. Evaluation of B-type natriuretic peptide for risk assessment in unstable angina/non-ST-elevation myocardial infarction: B-type natriuretic peptide and prognosis in TACTICS-TIMI 18. J Am Coll Cardiol 2003;41(8):1268; with permission.)

diagnosis of non–STE-ACS). Patients were followed concerning death for a median of 40 months. Compared with the lowest quartile, patients in the second, third, and fourth quartile had a relative risk (95% CI) of subsequent death of 4.2 (1.6–11.1), 10.7 (4.2–26.8), and 26.6 (10.8–65.5), respectively. The predictive value of NT-proBNP was evident in patients who had a final diagnosis of non–STE-ACS and in those who had other cardiac or noncardiac conditions (Fig. 3). Omland and colleagues [13] confirmed the strong independent association between the level of NT-proBNP and mortality, even when adjusted for age, Killip class, and LVEF determined by echocardiography.

Later the authors' group together with others reported the NT-proBNP substudy of the Global Use of Strategies to Open Ocluded Arteries IV (GUSTO-IV) trial [14], including 6809 patients who had non–STE-ACS. In this large cohort of patients, the associations between the NT-proBNP levels and other patient characteristics were clearly outlined. Higher levels of NT-proBNP were related to age, hypertension, diabetes, renal dysfunction, and previous history of cardiovascular disease. In the acute setting the level of NT-proBNP was related to the magnitude of myocardial damage (ie, level of troponin T) and inflammatory activity (ie, level of C-reactive protein [CRP]). Again, there was an increase in mortality with higher levels of NT-proBNP, with a significant separation of the survival curves already at 48 hours (mortality in lowest versus highest quartile: 0.2% versus 1.4%) and a continuing separation of the curves during the entire 1-year follow-up period. In fact, mortality increased exponentially throughout the entire range of NT-proBNP levels with a very low mortality of 0.4% in the lowest decile ($\leq$98 ng/L) and 27.1% in the highest decile (>4634 ng/L) (Fig. 4). The study also demonstrated that any elevation of NT-proBNP greater than the 97.5 percentile, 290 ng/L, in a healthy population matched for age and gender [16], was associated with an increased risk for death after the index event.

Unlike BNP, NT-proBNP is not cleaved by neutral endopeptidase and the elimination depends

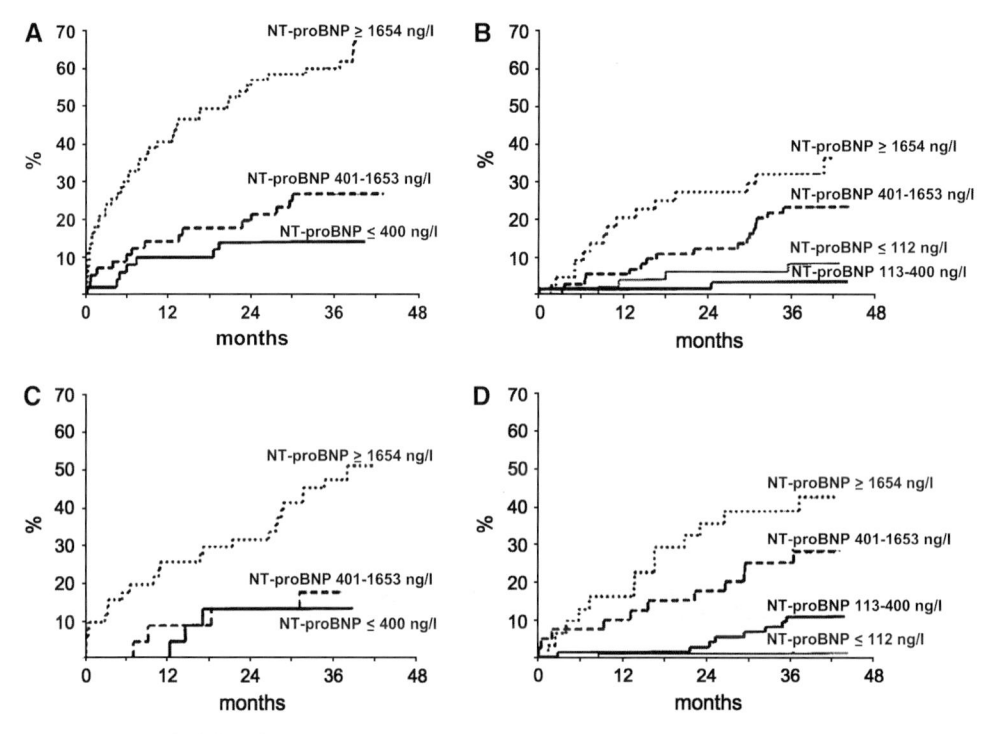

Fig. 3. Cumulative probability of death in patients who have (*A*) acute myocardial infarction (pooled log-rank, $P < .001$); (*B*) angina or unstable angina (pooled log-rank, $P < .001$); (*C*) other cardiac causes (pooled log-rank $P = .004$); (*D*) other noncardiac or unknown causes (pooled log-rank, $P < .001$). NT-proBNP, N-terminal pro brain natriuretic peptide. (*From* Jernberg T, Stridsberg M, Venge P, et al. N-terminal pro brain natriuretic peptide on admission for early risk stratification of patients with chest pain and no ST-segment elevation. J Am Coll Cardiol 2002;40(3):441; with permission.)

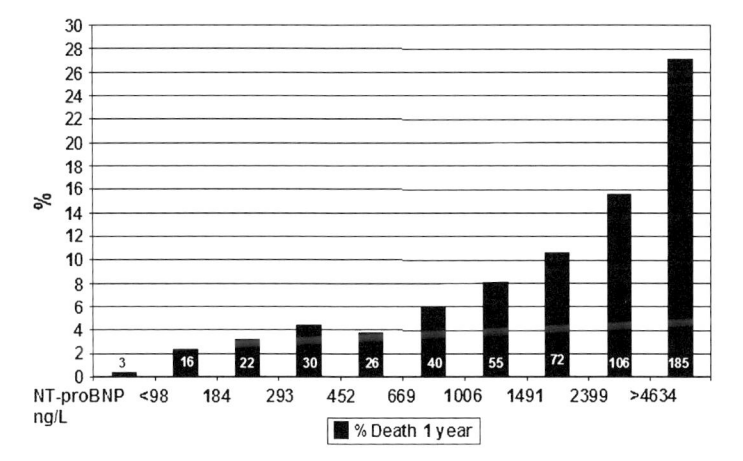

Fig. 4. Mortality at 1-year follow-up among strata of patients according to deciles of NT-proBNP levels. Number of deaths in each decile is given at the bottom of the bars. (*From* James SK, Lindahl B, Siegbahn A, et al. N-terminal pro-brain natriuretic peptide and other risk markers for the separate prediction of mortality and subsequent myocardial infarction in patients with unstable coronary artery disease: a Global Utilization of Strategies To Open Occluded Arteries (GUSTO)-IV substudy. Circulation 2003;108(3):278; with permission.)

on clearance by the kidneys. NT-proBNP levels therefore could potentially be less useful in patients who have renal insufficiency. NT-proBNP levels and creatinine clearance rates, however, provided independent and additive prognostic information on long-term mortality in the GUSTO-IV substudy [14]. Among patients in every quartile of creatinine clearance, mortality was increased with increasing quartiles of NT-proBNP (Fig. 5).

In univariable analysis, a higher level of NT-proBNP was also associated with a higher risk for future myocardial infarction (MI) in the GUSTO-IV substudy [14]. After adjustment for the multitude of covariates, however, there remained no

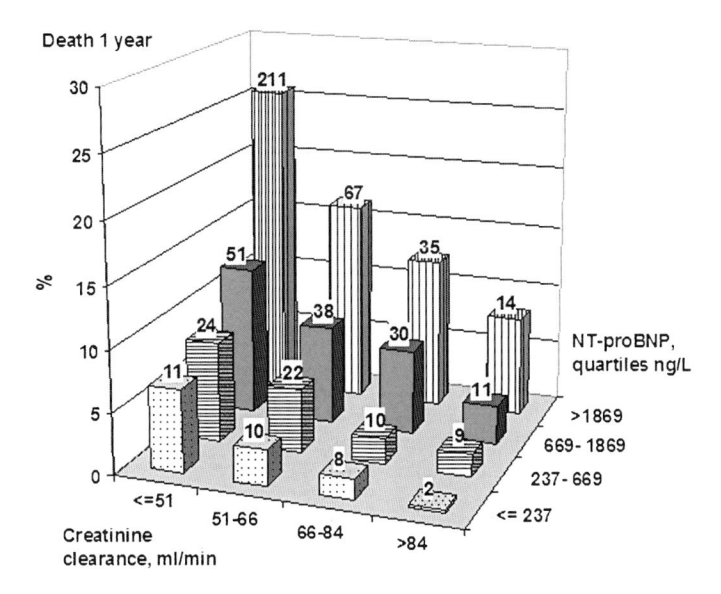

Fig. 5. Mortality at 1-year follow-up among strata of patients according to quartiles of NT-proBNP and quartiles of creatinine clearance. The number of deaths is given at the top of each bar. (*From* James SK, Lindahl B, Siegbahn A, et al. N-terminal pro-brain natriuretic peptide and other risk markers for the separate prediction of mortality and subsequent myocardial infarction in patients with unstable coronary artery disease: a Global Utilization of Strategies To Open Occluded Arteries (GUSTO)-IV substudy. Circulation 2003;108(3):280; with permission.)

independent association between the level of NT-proBNP and the risk for subsequent MI. The lack of independent association between natriuretic peptide level and risk for future MI might be explained by the fact that BNP and NT-proBNP levels are not related to processes that increase the likelihood of a new coronary plaque destabilization or formation of coronary thrombi. In contrast, BNP level has been shown to be associated with the risk for sudden death in patients who have heart failure [17]. An increased level of BNP or NT-proBNP thus may indicate an increased risk for ventricular arrhythmias, ventricular rupture, or terminal heart failure rather than MI.

Multimarker approach for early risk stratification of non–ST-elevation acute coronary syndromes

The number of different biochemical and other markers claimed to be useful for early risk assessment in non–STE-ACS is rapidly growing. It is important, however, not only to show that a new marker provides independent prognostic information, but also that the addition of the new marker provides *clinically meaningful* incremental information to what is already available from standard factors and markers, ie, the patient history, ECG changes, and troponin levels.

Sabatine and colleagues evaluated a multimarker approach combining troponin I, C-reactive protein, and BNP [18]. They found the combination useful for prediction of death and congestive heart failure, but the predictive power for MI was less impressive (Fig. 6), which is not surprising considering that neither C-reactive protein nor BNP has been shown to be predictive of MI alone. Bazzino and colleagues took another approach and evaluated the additive value of determination of NT-proBNP to the TIMI risk score (and ACC/AHA risk classification) (Fig. 7) [19]. The TIMI risk score is composed of information on five clinical variables, ST-segment changes, and level of a marker of myocardial necrosis. Elevation of NT-proBNP identified a group with a high risk of dying among the large group of patients classified to be at low risk with the TIMI risk score. Furthermore, the addition of NT-proBNP divided the group classified by TIMI risk score to be at intermediate risk to a group at low and high risk, respectively, whereas in the small group of patients found to be at high risk [20] by TIMI risk score, the NT-proBNP level did not add any clinically meaningful information.

NT-proBNP or BNP thus seems to be an attractive marker to incorporate in risk scores or risk assessment programs. More studies, however, in unselected chest pain populations and of the cost-effectiveness of incorporating NT-proBNP or BNP are needed before any firm recommendation can be made.

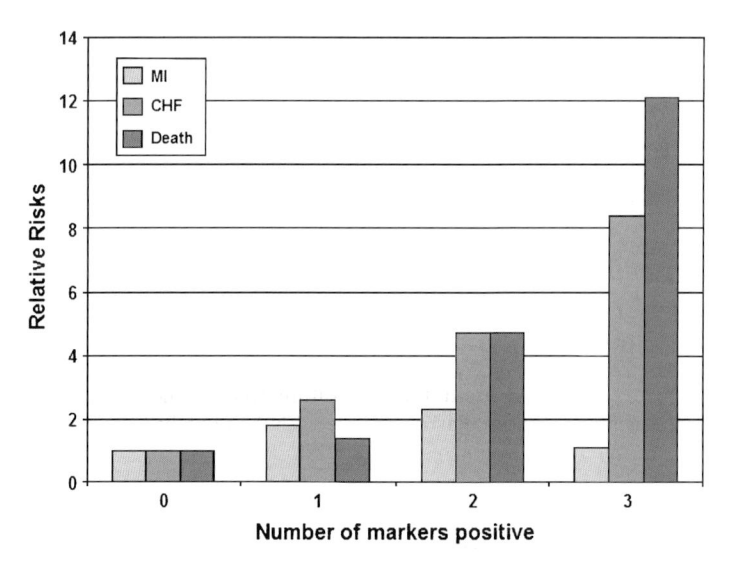

Fig. 6. Relative risks for a new MI, CHF, and death, respectively, according to number of markers (troponin I, C-reactive protein, and BNP) positive on admission. (*Data from* Sabatine MS, Morrow DA, de Lemos JA, et al. Multimarker approach to risk stratification in non-ST elevation acute coronary syndromes: simultaneous assessment of troponin I, C-reactive protein, and B-type natriuretic peptide. Circulation 2002;105(15):1760–3.)

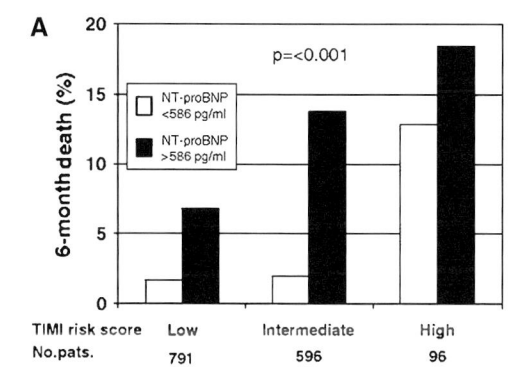

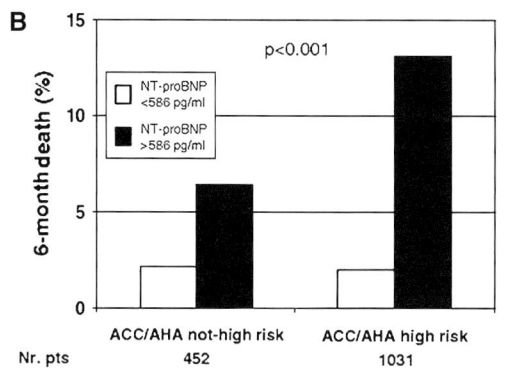

Fig. 7. (A) Six-month death rates among strata of patients according to NT-proBNP levels and TIMI risk categories (low, moderate, and high). (B) Six-month death rates among strata of patients according to NT-proBNP levels and ACC/AHA classification (non–high-risk and high risk). (From Bazzino O, Fuselli JJ, Botto F, et al. Relative value of N-terminal pro-brain natriuretic peptide, TIMI risk score, ACC/AHA prognostic classification and other risk markers in patients with non-ST-elevation acute coronary syndromes. Eur Heart J 2004;25(10):865; with permission.)

Selection of treatment in non–ST-elevation acute coronary syndromes

Although NT-proBNP and BNP are among the most powerful biomarkers for prediction of mortality in patients who have non–STE-ACS, there are only a few studies evaluating whether levels of BNP or NT-proBNP might be useful for selection of specific treatments, eg, revascularization. In the TACTICS-TIMI 18 trial [21], there was no appreciable difference in the reduction of death or MI by an invasive versus conservative strategy in those who had higher levels of BNP compared with those who had lower levels. The markers, however, do not predict the risk for future MI and the trial did not have the power to look at the reduction of mortality alone. Nevertheless, patients who had a BNP level greater than 80 ng/L tended to have a lower mortality after an invasive strategy, 7.9% versus 9.0%. On the contrary, in patients who had a BNP level less than 80 ng/L, the invasive strategy did not tend to decrease the overall low mortality, 1.9% versus 1.6% [11]. In the FRISC-2 trial [15], patients who had elevated NT-proBNP tended to have a greater survival benefit of an early invasive strategy compared with those who had lower NT-proBNP levels. An invasive strategy reduced the 2-year mortality by 3.6% from 10.8% to 7.2% (absolute risk reduction, 3.6%; $P = .11$) among patients who had NT-proBNP levels in the top tertile, whereas there was no effect in those who had lower levels of NT-proBNP. In the nonrandomized comparison of 30-day survivors in the GUSTO-IV trial, revascularization was associated with an absolute 1-year mortality reduction of 4.3% in patients who had a positive NT-proBNP [20]. In patients who had elevation of NT-proBNP greater than or equal to 237 ng/L, 1-year mortality thus was 2.7% versus 7.0% ($P < .001$) in patients who received versus did not receive revascularization. In patients who had NT-proBNP less than 237 ng/L, there was no difference in 1-year mortality between revascularized and non-revascularized patients (1.2% versus 1.2%). Troponin T and NT-proBNP seemed to stratify patients with versus without an improvement in outcome following revascularization. In a multivariable analysis also including a propensity score of receiving revascularization and the time-point of revascularization as a time-dependent variable, patients who had elevation of troponin-T and NT-proBNP, a significantly lower mortality after revascularization was observed (relative risk ratio (RR), 0.55; 95% CI, 0.4–0.7). On the contrary, revascularization was associated with a significant hazard in patients who had elevation of neither troponin T nor NT-proBNP (RR, 10.8; 95% CI, 2.1–56).

Although these data need to be confirmed in future studies, they suggest that BNP and NT-proBNP might be useful to identify those non–STE-ACS patients who would have a mortality benefit from an early invasive management. Whether patients who have non–STE-ACS and high levels of natriuretic peptides will obtain any specific benefit from intensified treatment with antithrombotics, beta-blockers, or angiotensin-converting enzyme inhibitors is still unknown.

ST-elevation myocardial infarction

Generally the prognostic value of biomarkers has been less studied in patients who have ST-elevated myocardial infarction (STEMI) than in patients who have non–STE-ACS. Elevation of troponin (T or I), however, on admission has been shown to be associated with an increased short- and long-term mortality in several large studies [22,23]. There are now also a limited number of studies showing that elevation of NT-proBNP or BNP is associated with increased mortality in STEMI in patients treated with fibrinolytics and primary percutaneous coronary intervention (PCI). The results of these studies are summarized in Table 3 [13,24–27]. NT-proBNP and BNP have remained as independent predictors of mortality in different multivariate models, for example, after adjustment for troponin level and clinical variables known to be important predictors of outcome (age, heart rate, blood pressure, and Killip class) [25] and after adjustment for age, LVEF, and Killip class [13]. Determination of troponin T and NT-proBNP on admission seem to give additive prognostic information (Fig. 8).

The levels of natriuretic peptides at admission increase by symptom duration [25,28], although the correlation was weak (r = 0.17) in the study of Björklund and colleagues [25]. Furthermore, the NT-proBNP/BNP level on admission has been found to be associated with heart rate, Killip class, and LVEF [13,25]. A weak association has also been found with the severity of CAD (coronary artery surgery study score [CASS]) [25]. NT-proBNP measured after 24 hours correlated significantly with measures of infarct size in one study [28].

Whether determination of NT-proBNP/BNP in STEMI is useful for selection of treatment is unknown. There are no published studies in STEMI patients evaluating whether the effect of a particular treatment differs in relation to levels of NT-proBNP/BNP.

Special issues

NT-proBNP or BNP

NT-proBNP and BNP are released in a 1:1 fashion. Because of the difference in plasma half-life and elimination, however, the concentrations of the two peptides in plasma are different. Nevertheless, the levels of the two markers are closely correlated [5]. The only published study with a head-to-head comparison between the two peptides in ACS regarding outcome concluded that BNP and NT-proBNP were equivalent prognostic markers [29], and the same conclusion was drawn in a study comparing the prognostic value of the two markers in stable angina [5]. There is thus currently no scientific evidence to support a recommendation of one marker over the other for evaluation of prognosis in IHD.

Choice of appropriate cut-off values

A single cut-off value of a biochemical marker is convenient to use in clinical practice and in decision algorithms. Regarding the natriuretic peptides, however, using one single cut-off might be an oversimplification, considering the nature of the natriuretic peptides and the continuous increase of risk associated with increasing levels.

One important issue is whether cut-off values should be related to age and gender. It is well known that BNP and NT-proBNP levels increase with age and are higher in women. The reasons for the sex-related difference are still unclear. That the age-related mortality is lower in women than in men, however, suggests that the reason for this gender difference does not cause increased mortality. The authors suggest, therefore, that gender differences should be considered when determining suitable cut-off values, especially to identify low-risk patients. Because the higher levels of BNP and NT-proBNP found in elderly patients are presumably explained by a higher

Table 3
Association between outcome and NT-proBNP/BNP levels in ST-elevation myocardial infarction

Study	Endpoint	N	Marker	F-U	Cut-off	Adjusted OR or HR (95% CI)	
[24]	Death	126	BNP	42 d	100 ng/L		16.3 (1.4–187)
[25]	Death	782	NT-proBNP	1 y	—	1 SD increase	2.3 (1.3–3.9)
[26]	Death	615	NT-proBNP	30 d	Quartiles	4th vs. 1st	approx. 7[a]
[27]	Death	88	BNP	30 d	Quartiles	4th vs. 1st	5.6 (1.6–20.5)[b]
[13]	Death	204	NT-proBNP	51 m	Median		2.6 (0.7–8.8)

Abbreviations: CI, confidence interval; F-U, follow-up time; HR, hazard ratio; N, number of patients; OR, odds ratio.
[a] Estimated from Fig. 4 in [26].
[b] Unadjusted.

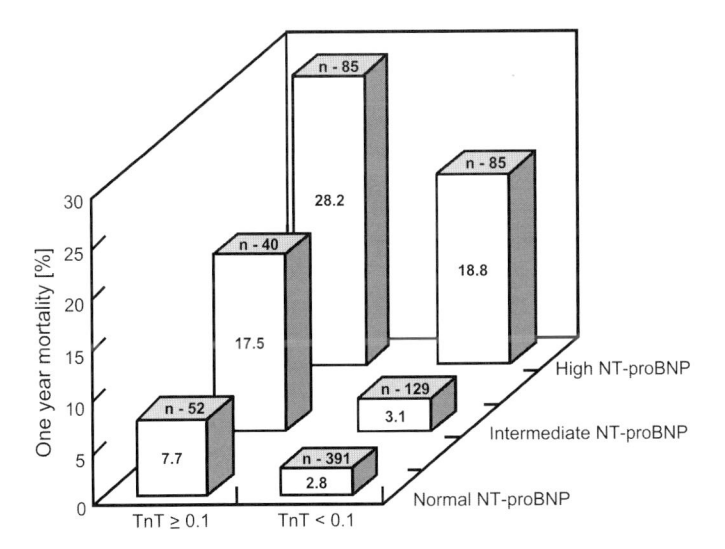

Fig. 8. One-year mortality according to the combination of NT-proBNP (ng/L) and TnT (μg/L) in STEMI patients. (*From* Bjorklund E, Jernberg T, Johanson P, et al. Admission N-terminal pro-brain natriuretic peptide and its interaction with admission troponin T and ST segment resolution for early risk stratification in ST elevation myocardial infarction. Heart 2006;92(6):738; with permission.)

prevalence of subclinical cardiac conditions [30], however, age-dependent cut-off values might not be necessary when using these methods for risk stratification.

One important task in managing patients who have a suspicion of an ACS is to identify low-risk patients. By virtue of being unspecific markers of reduced cardiac performance, the natriuretic peptides are useful for that purpose and the upper reference level in a healthy population seems to be an appropriate cut-off. Cut-off values less than the upper reference value would lead to unacceptably low specificities. Conversely, patients who have elevated levels of NT-proBNP or BNP are at increased risk for a fatal complication that may merit further investigation and treatment. A cut-off value to identify the high-risk group, with a probably greater benefit from a more aggressive treatment strategy (including early revascularization), is difficult to define from the literature and tends to be somewhat arbitrary. In fact, mortality increases with increasing levels of NT-proBNP and BNP, and no obvious high-risk cut-off can be chosen. It is important for clinicians to recognize that the risk is different for a patient who has a level of the natriuretic peptide just higher than the upper reference level compared with a patient who has a level 10 times the upper reference level, although both patients are "positive" for that marker (see Fig. 4).

According to the authors' data, the 97.5 percentile values for NT-proBNP in men and women younger than 65 years of age can be approximated to be 200 ng/L and 300 ng/L, whereas these values are somewhat higher in those older than 65 years of age (approximately 300 ng/L for men and 400 ng/L for women) [16].

For BNP, the reference values differ between assays and studies and there is a lack of standardization [31,32]. For BNP determined by the Biosite assay, however, an empirically defined, single cut-off value of 80 ng/L rather than the upper reference level has been suggested [10,11].

When should NT-proBNP/BNP be measured in acute coronary syndromes?

When the natriuretic peptides should be measured in ACS depends of course on the clinical question. To be able to make a risk assessment that can guide the initial therapy and management, it is important to have the necessary information available as soon as possible. In the study of Jernberg and colleagues [12], NT-proBNP levels on admission gave identical prognostic information as levels obtained 6 hours after admission and the relative change in levels between the two time points did not provide any extra information. The study of Heescen and colleagues [33], however, indicates that dynamic changes are of importance. Patients who had low values of NT-proBNP on admission that increased and became elevated at 72 hours had a high risk for future events, and conversely, patients who had high values on admission that decreased and were normalized at 72 hours had a low risk. Further studies hence are needed to establish whether a second sample in addition to the admissions sample adds clinically relevant information, and if so, when it should be obtained.

Summary

Levels of the natriuretic peptides NT-proBNP and BNP are independently associated with mortality in the entire spectrum of ischemic heart disease. Measurement of NT-proBNP or BNP, in addition to standard variables currently used for risk assessment, seems to add clinically relevant, incremental prognostic information regarding mortality. The natriuretic peptides, however, are not independently predictive of AMI. Because long-term mortality increases with increasing levels of NT-proBNP and BNP, an important, unresolved issue that needs further research is to define optimal cut-off levels for different clinical questions.

Although there is some evidence suggesting that measurements of NT-proBNP or BNP might be useful for selection of therapy in ACS, this important issue also needs further investigation.

References

[1] Kragelund C, Gronning B, Kober L, et al. N-terminal pro-B-type natriuretic peptide and long-term mortality in stable coronary heart disease. N Engl J Med 2005;352(7):666–75.

[2] Ndrepepa G, Braun S, Niemoller K, et al. Prognostic value of N-terminal pro-brain natriuretic peptide in patients with chronic stable angina. Circulation 2005;112(14):2102–7.

[3] Saleh N, Braunschweig F, Jensen J, et al. Usefulness of preprocedural serum N-terminal pro-brain natriuretic peptide levels to predict long-term outcome after percutaneous coronary intervention in patients with normal troponin T levels. Am J Cardiol 2006; 97(6):830–4.

[4] Schnabel R, Rupprecht HJ, Lackner KJ, et al. Analysis of N-terminal-pro-brain natriuretic peptide and C-reactive protein for risk stratification in stable and unstable coronary artery disease: results from the AtheroGene study. Eur Heart J 2005;26(3):241–9.

[5] Richards M, Nicholls M, Espiner E, et al. Comparison of B-type natriuretic peptides for assessment of cardiac function and prognosis in stable ischemic heart disease. J Am Coll Cardiol 2006;47(1): 52–60.

[6] Omland T, Richards A, Wergeland R, et al. B-type natriuretic peptide and long-term survival in patients with stable coronary artery disease. Am J Cardiol 2005;95(1):24–8.

[7] Schnabel R, Lubos E, Rupprecht H, et al. B-type natriuretic peptide and the risk of cardiovascular events and death in patients with stable angina: results from the AtheroGene Study. J Am Coll Cardiol 2005;47(3):552–8.

[8] Kragelund C, Gronning B, Omland T, et al. Is N-terminal pro B-type natriuretic peptide (NT-proBNP) a useful screening test for angiographic findings in patients with stable coronary disease? Am Heart J 2006;151(3):712.e711–17.

[9] Ndrepepa G, Braun S, Mehilli J, et al. Plasma levels of N-terminal pro-brain natriuretic peptide in patients with coronary artery disease and relation to clinical presentation, angiographic severity, and left ventricular ejection fraction. Am J Cardiol 2005;95(5):553–7.

[10] de Lemos JA, Morrow DA, Bentley JH, et al. The prognostic value of B-type natriuretic peptide in patients with acute coronary syndromes. N Engl J Med 2001;345(14):1014–21.

[11] Morrow DA, de Lemos JA, Sabatine MS, et al. Evaluation of B-type natriuretic peptide for risk assessment in unstable angina/non-ST-elevation myocardial infarction: B-type natriuretic peptide and prognosis in TACTICS-TIMI 18 [erratum]. J Am Coll Cardiol 2003;41(10):1852.

[12] Jernberg T, Stridsberg M, Venge P, et al. N-terminal pro brain natriuretic peptide on admission for early risk stratification of patients with chest pain and no ST-segment elevation. J Am Coll Cardiol 2002; 40(3):437–45.

[13] Omland T, Persson A, Ng L, et al. N-terminal pro-B-type natriuretic peptide and long-term mortality in acute coronary syndromes. Circulation 2002; 106(23):2913–8.

[14] James SK, Lindahl B, Siegbahn A, et al. N-terminal pro-brain natriuretic peptide and other risk markers for the separate prediction of mortality and subsequent myocardial infarction in patients with unstable coronary artery disease: a Global Utilization of Strategies To Open Occluded Arteries (GUSTO)-IV substudy. Circulation 2003; 108(3):275–81.

[15] Jernberg T, Lindahl B, Siegbahn A, et al. N-terminal pro-brain natriuretic peptide in relation to inflammation, myocardial necrosis, and the effect of an invasive strategy in unstable coronary artery disease. J Am Coll Cardiol 2003;42(11):1909–16.

[16] Johnston N, Jernberg T, Lindahl B, et al. Biochemical indicators of cardiac and renal function in a healthy elderly population. Clin Biochem 2004; 37(3):210–6.

[17] Berger R, Huelsman M, Strecker K, et al. B-type natriuretic peptide predicts sudden death in patients with chronic heart failure. Circulation 2002; 105(20):2392–7.

[18] Sabatine MS, Morrow DA, de Lemos JA, et al. Multimarker approach to risk stratification in non-ST elevation acute coronary syndromes: simultaneous assessment of troponin I, C-reactive protein, and B-type natriuretic peptide. Circulation 2002;105(15): 1760–3.

[19] Bazzino O, Fuselli JJ, Botto F, et al. Relative value of N-terminal pro-brain natriuretic peptide, TIMI risk score, ACC/AHA prognostic classification and other risk markers in patients with non-ST-elevation acute coronary syndromes. Eur Heart J 2004;25(10): 859–66.

[20] James S, Lindahl B, Lindback J, et al. Troponin T and N-terminal pro B-type natriuretic peptide predict mortality benefit from coronary revascularization in acute coronary syndromes—a GUSTO IV substudy. J Am Coll Cardiol 2006; in press.

[21] Morrow DA, de Lemos JA, Sabatine MS, et al. Evaluation of B-type natriuretic peptide for risk assessment in unstable angina/non-ST-elevation myocardial infarction: B-type natriuretic peptide and prognosis in TACTICS-TIMI 18. J Am Coll Cardiol 2003;41(8): 1264–72.

[22] Stubbs P, Collinson P, Moseley D, et al. Prognostic significance of admission troponin T concentrations in patients with myocardial infarction. Circulation 1996;94(6):1291–7.

[23] Ohman EM, Armstrong PW, White HD, et al. Risk stratification with a point-of-care cardiac troponin T test in acute myocardial infarction. GUSTO III Investigators. Global use of strategies to open occluded coronary arteries. Am J Cardiol 1999; 84(11):1281–6.

[24] Grabowski M, Filipiak KJ, Karpinski G, et al. Serum B-type natriuretic peptide levels on admission predict not only short-term death but also angiographic success of procedure in patients with acute ST-elevation myocardial infarction treated with primary angioplasty. Am Heart J 2004;148(4): 655–62.

[25] Bjorklund E, Jernberg T, Johanson P, et al. Admission N-terminal pro-brain natriuretic peptide and its interaction with admission troponin T and ST segment resolution for early risk stratification in ST elevation myocardial infarction. Heart 2006;92(6): 735–40.

[26] Galvani M, Ferrini D, Ottani F. Natriuretic peptides for risk stratification of patients with acute coronary syndromes. Eur J Heart Fail 2004;6(3):327–33.

[27] Grabowski M, Filipiak KJ, Karpinski G, et al. Prognostic value of B-type natriuretic peptide levels on admission in patients with acute ST elevation myocardial infarction. Acta Cardiol 2005;60(5):537–42.

[28] Ezekowitz JA, Theroux P, Chang W, et al. N-terminal pro-brain natriuretic peptide and the timing, extent and mortality in ST elevation myocardial infarction. Can J Cardiol 2006;22(5):393–7.

[29] Richards AM, Nicholls MG, Espiner EA, et al. B-type natriuretic peptides and ejection fraction for prognosis after myocardial infarction. Circulation 2003;107(22):2786–92.

[30] Sayama H, Nakamura Y, Saito N, et al. Why is the concentration of plasma brain natriuretic peptide in elderly inpatients greater than normal? Coron Artery Dis 1999;10(7):537–40.

[31] Wang TJ, Larson MG, Levy D, et al. Impact of age and sex on plasma natriuretic peptide levels in healthy adults. Am J Cardiol 2002;90(3):254–8.

[32] Redfield MM, Rodeheffer RJ, Jacobsen SJ, et al. Plasma brain natriuretic peptide concentration: impact of age and gender. J Am Coll Cardiol 2002; 40(5):976–82.

[33] Heeschen C, Hamm CW, Mitrovic V, et al, for the Platelet Receptor Inhibition in Ischemic Syndrome Management I. N-terminal pro-B-type natriuretic peptide levels for dynamic risk stratification of patients with acute coronary syndromes. Circulation 2004;110(20):3206–12.

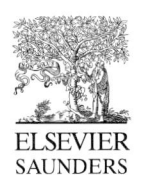

Natriuretic Peptides in Screening for Cardiac Dysfunction

W.H. Wilson Tang, MD*

Cleveland Clinic, Cleveland, OH, USA

The clinical syndrome of heart failure is a devastating and costly disease. It is believed to progress in at-risk patients (stage A) from a preclinical, asymptomatic stage with demonstrable heart muscle abnormalities (stage B), to an overt symptomatic heart failure syndrome (stages C and D) [1]. Therefore, to address the accruing morbidity and mortality and the increasing cost of advanced heart failure, effective screening strategies are needed desperately to identify the estimated 8 to 10 million asymptomatic patients who have evident structural heart abnormalities before overt symptoms ensue. Large-scale epidemiologic studies consistently have established that the prevalence of "stage B heart failure" is at least equal to the prevalence of symptomatic heart failure [2]. This indicates that a substantial population is at risk for disease progression. These data laid the foundation for the concept that early identification and treatment of factors (pharmacologic and nonpharmacologic) that lead to myocardial dysfunction may abrogate progression to symptomatic advanced heart failure.

The diagnostic usefulness of B-type natriuretic peptide (BNP) and aminoterminal-proBNP (NT-proBNP) in the acute setting prompted interest in the evaluation of these clinically available biomarkers as effective screening tools; however, there are several "prerequisites" for a suitable biomarker for screening of cardiac dysfunction that were summarized recently (Table 1) [3].

This article outlines the challenges for natriuretic peptide screening for left ventricular systolic dysfunction (LVSD). In addition, it reviews the concept of optimal screening strategies based on cost-effectiveness analyses, and examines recent data regarding the usefulness of natriuretic screening for specific patient populations.

Challenges in natriuretic peptide screening

There are several important, but challenging, limitations of the existing literature. First and foremost, after individuals who have stage B heart failure have been identified, the optimal methods and impact of serial monitoring and targeted therapy remain largely unknown. Current data regarding the benefits of early interventions (eg, angiotensin-converting enzyme inhibitor therapy) are implied from earlier work. Medical interventions (eg, diuretics and β-adrenergic blockers) can affect plasma natriuretic peptide levels, and interpretation of single time-point evaluations in patients using such agents may be complicated [4].

Screening studies using natriuretic peptides have been limited to observational study designs, either from large-scale, population-based epidemiologic studies, or single- or multi-center prospective cohort studies. Plasma natriuretic peptides generally increase with worsening systolic and diastolic dysfunction in men and women (Fig. 1); however, cut-off values usually are determined retrospectively and the decision statistics are determined post hoc. Furthermore, cut-off values may be specific to the assays used as well as to the type of dysfunction (systolic or diastolic dysfunction) that is being detected, and there is no harmonization among the different commercially

---

* Section of Heart Failure and Cardiac Transplantation Medicine, Department of Cardiovascular Medicine, Cleveland Clinic, 9500 Euclid Avenue, Desk F25, Cleveland, OH 44195.
 E-mail address: tangw@ccf.org

Table 1
Prerequisites for population screening: cardiac dysfunction as case study

Concept	Case for natriuretic peptides
The condition is of public health importance	Cardiac dysfunction and heart failure are prevalent and portend poor prognosis
The natural history is understood, and there is an unsuspected, but detectable, preclinical stage	The progression from cardiac dysfunction to overt heart failure has been well documented, although the pace and characteristics may vary
There is an ethical, acceptable, safe, and accurate screening test for early detection and intervention	Natriuretic peptide testing and echocardiography are minimally invasive techniques for detecting cardiac dysfunction
Consensus is reached on the frequency, screening ages, quality control and monitoring of screening program, and mechanisms of referral and treatment of positive tests	Cost-effective screening is only applicable in patients with higher ($>1\%$) prevalence, and current evidence support screening in elderly men and patients who have had a myocardial infarction
There is sufficient political will, resources, and strategies to adopt and implement screening practice	There are initiatives in the postinfarction population based on the need to identify patients who do not have overt symptoms but who have impaired cardiac function (LVEF $\leq 30\%$) for implantable cardioverter defibrillators, but no population-based advocacy for screening

available assays. Because of the morbidity and mortality of the condition, it is not ethical to withhold the findings or start treatment once cardiac dysfunction is detected. Therefore, a randomized study is difficult to conduct, unless the "gold standard" reaches beyond simply detecting cardiac dysfunction to improving clinical events. No study has embarked on completing this ambitious aim, despite the fact that most studies have linked elevated BNP or NT-proBNP with higher

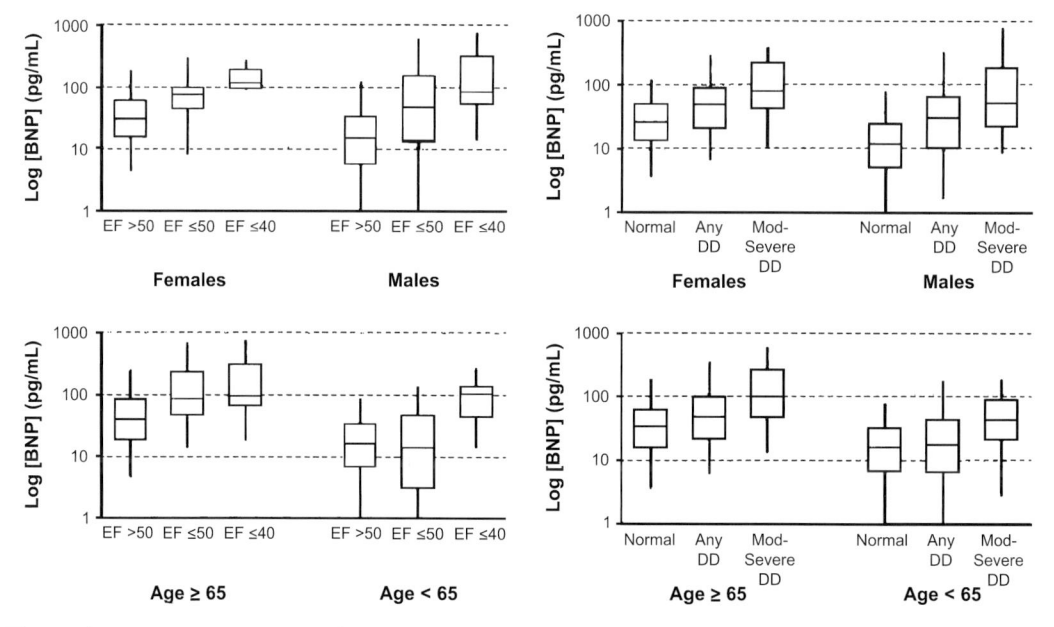

Fig. 1. Plasma BNP levels to screen for patients who have LVSD. EF, ejection fraction; DD, diastolic dysfunction. (*From* Redfield MM, Rodeheffer RJ, Jacobsen SJ, et al. Plasma brain natriuretic peptide to detect preclinical ventricular systolic or diastolic dysfunction: a community-based study. Circulation 2004;109(25):3178; with permission.)

mortality and morbidity. Three variables that need further discussion include biologic variability, assay variability, and target definition variability.

Biologic variability

The use of natriuretic peptides as screening biomarkers for heart failure is promising because of their good specificity in the setting of overt heart failure; however, it is clear from early investigations that BNP and NT-proBNP levels have wide intra- and interindividual biologic variability, and their levels are dependent on the clinical setting [5]. Load-independent variations of natriuretic peptide expression may confound the ability to detect subclinical cardiac dysfunction [6]. Natriuretic peptide levels vary with age and gender [7–9], as well as with body habitus. Some studies used age- and gender-specific cut-offs, which would make it less ideal and complicated for broad adoption. Also, the accuracy of natriuretic peptides may be less robust in at-risk patients in whom differences between normal or abnormal may be small in absolute values. A simple explanation for this phenomenon may be the fact that most asymptomatic patients are well compensated, often with relatively normal wall stress and intracardiac pressures.

Assay variability

Different clinically available natriuretic peptide assays may have different performance characteristics, and may report different numerical values of BNP or NT-proBNP for the same blood sample. For example, different assays that measure BNP may have different sensitivities when using the same "cut-off" [10]. Although this variation may not affect the overall diagnostic accuracy for detecting acute heart failure, the need to have a specific optimal "cut-off" for each assay for screening purposes may complicate the broad adoption of population-wide screening, particularly when most epidemiologic studies used research-based assays (eg, Shionogi). In general, the cut-off values that are derived from one study that used research-based assays can be difficult to convert directly into values that are appropriate for clinically available assays.

Target definition variability

Most clinical investigations of BNP or NT-proBNP screening in the general population have had limited ability to detect individuals who have marginally impaired left ventricular abnormalities. This may be due to the nonspecific association between plasma BNP and NT-proBNP levels and LVSD in the lower range of the assay values. The definition of left ventricular systolic function is prone to errors in measurements (often ± 5% by echocardiography), and it may vary with imaging modalities (eg, average left ventricular ejection fraction [LVEF] derived from radionuclide ventriculography can be 5%–10% higher than that derived from echocardiography). Nevertheless, the overall data suggest that plasma BNP and NT-proBNP testing are able to detect more severe LVSD (LVEF ≤ 30%) better than borderline systolic dysfunction (LVEF 40%–50%). This may have important implications regarding the initiation of therapy and risk stratification.

Defining optimal screening strategies: cost-effectiveness considerations

One of the most contentious debates regarding the use of natriuretic peptides in screening is the issue of cost-effectiveness. In the general context of public health, few screening modalities in preventive medicine can achieve true cost-effectiveness, because the "benefit" part of the cost/benefit ratio often is subjective, and it largely can be dependent on the societal point of view and can be enforced by strong political will. Nevertheless, there have been some data regarding the cost-effectiveness of using natriuretic peptide screening. The consensus is that population-based screening can be cost-effective when focused on high-risk populations that have a greater prevalence of LVSD.

In a retrospective analysis, Nielsen and colleagues [11] evaluated a random sample of 1,257 community subjects (age 25–74 years) that were divided into three risk groups: (1) symptomatic ischemic heart disease (n = 140); (2) blood pressure greater than 160/95 mm Hg or an abnormal electrocardiogram (high risk, n = 269); and (3) none of these risk factors (low risk, n = 823). The prevalence of LVSD was 19%, 6%, and 0.7%, respectively. Raised BNP concentrations (>8 pg/mL) using their in-house assay occurred in 71%, 64%, and 41%, respectively, all with acceptable sensitivities (95.1%, 99.0%, and 99.8% respectively). Screening only high-risk subjects with BNP before echocardiography could have reduced the cost per detected case of LVSD by 26% for the cost ratio of 1/20 (BNP/echocardiogram).

Heidenreich and colleagues [12] performed a meticulous cost-benefit analysis by stratifying several scenarios based on the concomitant use of echocardiography, a standard "cut-off" value for BNP, and the initiation of angiotensin-converting enzyme inhibitors for the "positive" cases based on assumptions from the SOLVD-Prevention data from 2 decades ago. The main findings were twofold: (1) cost-effectiveness using BNP testing only can be achieved when the overall prevalence of heart failure is at least 1%, and, therefore, it may not be useful in women in whom the prevalence may be too low; and (2) BNP testing every 3 years for men who are older than 60 years (estimated prevalence of LVSD ≥ 1%) may achieve an acceptable less than $50,000/quality adjusted life-year gained. These analyses probably will be challenged with changes in the assumptions following technologic advances as portable echocardiography becomes more affordable and more widely accepted in noncardiology specialties.

Population screening for cardiac dysfunction using natriuretic peptides

Several published studies evaluated the use of natriuretic peptide screening in detecting cardiac dysfunction in an unselected general population. Most of the data are derived from large epidemiology studies that used research-based assays, although the same trends are present in validation studies that were performed with clinically available assays. Table 2 outlines the decision statistics of detecting cardiac dysfunction using natriuretic peptides. Diagnostic accuracies and reliability can be enhanced greatly by targeting specific high-risk populations (eg, the elderly) or after the definitions of cardiac dysfunction are optimized [13]. Nevertheless, natriuretic peptides provide independent prognostic values beyond LVEF in the screening population [14]. Combining data from three large-scale European epidemiologic studies, McDonagh and colleagues [15] explored the role of NT-proBNP in screening for cardiac dysfunction. Using age- and gender-specific cut-off values in a population of 3,051 individuals (aged 25–89 years) with a 3.1% prevalence of heart failure and 10% incidence of cardiac dysfunction, the investigators found that abnormal NT-proBNP levels can be explained by heart failure that is due to underlying LVSD in 30% of cases, but it can be explained by structural heart disease or renal insufficiency in 64% of patients. Similar conclusions regarding the detection of "abnormalities" have been drawn from other populations, especially when BNP data are combined with electrocardiograms and history of ischemic heart diseases [16–18].

The use of urinary N-terminal BNP measurements parallels the results that are obtained from measuring plasma N-terminal BNP levels. Recently, a research-based urinary NT-proBNP assay demonstrated excellent concordance and reliability with plasma BNP and NT-proBNP levels with respect to diagnostic accuracy (Fig. 2) [19]. These results need to be reproduced using clinically available assays.

Table 2
Epidemiological studies demonstrating the accuracy of utilizing natriuretic peptide screening in the general population

Study	n	Definition	Limit (pg/ml)	Sens	Spec	ROC
Vasan et al [79]	1,470 (M)	FS < 29%	>21	53%	84%	.72
	1,707 (F)			26%	89%	.56
Costello-Boerrigter et al [80]	1,869	EF ≤ 40%	228 (N-BNP)	87%	86%	.94
	479	FS < 28%	66 (BNP)	81%	81%	.81
Luchner et al [81]	126	Visual	>34	28%	86%	.61
Landray et al [82]	155	Visual	>17.9	88%	34%	–
Smith et al [83]	1,252	EF ≤ 30%	>64.7	92%	65%	.85
McDonagh et al [13]	466	EF < 45%	>17.9	77%	87%	.88
Yamamoto et al [84]	400	EF < 50%	>37	79%	64%	.79
Krishnaswamy et al [85]	254	EF ≤ 45%	>87	90%	67%	.82
Omland et al [86]	1,360	EF ≤ 45%	"Positive"	–	–	.74
Ng et al [87]			>19.2	–	44%	.94

Abbreviations: BNP, B-type natriuretic peptide; EF, ejection fraction; F, female; FS, fractional shortening; M, male; N-BNP, aminoterminal pro-B-type natriuretic peptide; ROC, receiver operator characteristic; Sens, sensitivity; Spec, specificity.

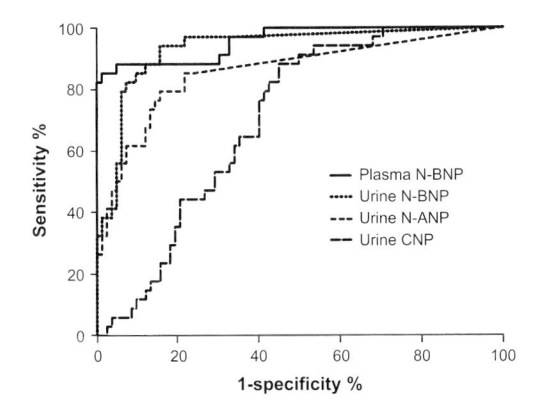

Fig. 2. Receiver operator characteristics curves for detecting LVSD using plasma and urine natriuretic peptides. N-ANP, aminoterminal A-type natriuretic peptide; N-BNP, aminoterminal B-type natriuretic peptide; CNP, C-type natriuretic peptide. (*From* Ng LL, Geeranavar S, Jennings SC, et al. Diagnosis of heart failure using urinary natriuretic peptides. Clin Sci 2004;106:132; with permission. © Copyright 2004, The Biochemical Society.)

Newer approaches that use multimarker strategies also are being developed. Ng and colleagues [20] found that the addition of plasma myeloperoxidase and high-sensitivity C-reactive protein to natriuretic screening improved diagnostic accuracy for detection of LVSD in a general population. The cut-off values were determined in a post hoc fashion using research-based assays, however, and direct translation to commercially available assays and validation of their predictive values requires further studies.

Specific at-risk patient populations

In general, because of the low prevalence of asymptomatic disease conditions in the general population, screening often is performed in individuals who are at risk for developing a particular disease. This "at-risk" population (or stage A heart failure) includes patients who have a history of coronary artery disease (especially with a history of myocardial infarction), diabetes mellitus, poorly controlled (stages I and II) hypertension, family history of cardiomyopathy, or previous cytotoxic chemotherapy treatment [1]. The prevalence of stage A heart failure and the relative risk for developing heart failure in the "at-risk" population remain unclear, however. In a hospital-based echocardiographic screening study, Baker and colleagues [21] identified consecutive patients who did not have heart failure but who did have a history of myocardial infarction, coronary artery disease, diabetes mellitus, and hypertension and had echocardiographic evidence of LVSD (prevalence of 15%, 13%, 7%, and 5%, respectively) when screened routinely using limited echocardiography dysfunction. Routine screening with natriuretic peptides in the elderly population also has been debated [22], and the latest guidelines still do not support routine screening with the current level of clinical evidence [1].

Patients who have myocardial infarction

Plasma BNP and NT-proBNP are considered to be useful in the setting of acute myocardial infarction (MI) in the absence of overt heart failure, where plasma BNP levels have been associated inversely with post-MI LVEF. Some of the earliest work led by Richards and colleagues [23–25] demonstrated the robust diagnostic and prognostic role of BNP and NT-proBNP in this setting, synergistic with LVEF and other biomarkers. In plasma, early plasma BNP concentrations that were less than twofold the upper limit of normal (20 pmol/L) using the Christchurch assay had 100% negative predictive value for LVEF of less than 40% at 3 to 5 months after infarction [23].

There are several specific issues regarding the use of BNP and NT-proBNP for screening in the post-MI setting. Meticulous serial assessment of natriuretic peptide revealed that the accuracy of BNP screening is variable as a result of heterogeneity in the patterns of increase and decrease of plasma levels over time, in various study populations, and in the timing of sampling. As such, echocardiography probably will remain the main method of assessing left ventricular structural and functional abnormalities after an MI, particular when indications for specific therapy (eg, aldosterone receptor antagonists, implantable cardioverter defibrillator) are based on identification of impaired LVEF.

Patients who have diabetes mellitus

Cardiovascular disease is the leading cause of death in patients who have diabetes mellitus. Attempts to improve this statistic tend to focus primarily on the prevention of coronary artery disease; however, coronary artery disease is not the sole cause of cardiac death in diabetic patients. There has been considerable interest in considering BNP or NT-proBNP screening in patients who have diabetes mellitus, because heart failure and structural abnormalities (including a unique entity called "diabetic cardiomyopathy") are prevalent in this population [26]. There also is a recognized progression of cardiac dysfunction over time [27], particularly in those with poor glycemic control [28]. Incident development of heart failure has been associated with significant mortality in patients who have diabetes mellitus [29]. Therefore, prescreening diabetic patients with plasma BNP or NT-proBNP may permit identification of individuals who are likely to have left ventricular abnormalities so that they may be referred for echocardiography and receive targeted therapy.

Overall, the data regarding screening for cardiac dysfunction in patients who have diabetes mellitus have been mixed. Some studies found that elevated natriuretic peptide levels in asymptomatic diabetic patients may indicate underlying cardiac dysfunction [30,31], whereas others have questioned their usefulness [32,33]. Nevertheless, elevated natriuretic peptide levels have been associated with autonomic dysfunction and microvascular abnormalities, and, therefore, remain good prognostic markers [34,35]. Obesity may be an important confounder; in the general population, there is an inverse relationship between body mass index and natriuretic peptide levels [36].

Patients who have renal insufficiency

The challenge of using natriuretic peptides to detect cardiac dysfunction is compounded with the confounders of impaired renal clearance, large volume shifts (especially in the population that is on dialysis), and the inverse relationship with hemoglobin levels that can increase natriuretic peptide levels [37–39]. Patients who had chronic kidney disease and elevated natriuretic peptides had an increased risk for subsequent coronary events as well as underlying left ventricular hypertrophy in those who were not [40,41] and were [42] on dialysis. Meanwhile, the reduction in the ratio between BNP and NT-proBNP seemed to be higher in patients who were on dialysis and had underlying LVSD [43]. Nevertheless, the clinical usefulness is still highly debated as a result of the many confounding factors that contribute to the exact levels at a single time-point [44].

Patients who are undergoing chemotherapy

Patients who are undergoing cancer chemotherapy with drugs that can be detrimental to cardiac function (eg, anthracyclines) pose a unique situation whereby cardiac dysfunction can be anticipated, even in the most careful drug titration and monitoring schedules. Plasma BNP levels are elevated following anthracycline administration [45]. Patients who have preserved cardiac function by baseline echocardiogram and elevated plasma BNP levels also may have an increased risk for the development of cardiac dysfunction; however, studies have been small, and evidence to support the routine use of BNP for screening purposes is lacking. This will be a particularly significant problem with the development of tyrosine kinase inhibitors with which cardiotoxicity was observed in clinical trials, and likely will be more widespread than considered previously. The difficulty is to balance the dramatic benefits of these compounds with the potential cardiac risks; the importance of cardiac screening and monitoring will be paramount.

Patients who have hypertension

Increased left ventricular mass and asymptomatic LVSD and left ventricular diastolic dysfunction are the remodeling phenotypes that are found commonly in patients who have poorly controlled hypertension that could be considered for population-wide screening. There is substantial variability in natriuretic peptide levels [46], however; although combining BNP and C-reactive protein may provide good negative predictive value to exclude potentially the presence of underlying structural heart disease [47]. In the Losartan Intervention for Endpoint reduction in hypertension (LIFE) trial, treatment with losartan and atenolol was associated with a reduction in left ventricular mass, as well as a corresponding reduction in plasma BNP levels [48]. The ability of plasma BNP and aminoterminal pro-A-type natriuretic peptide (NT-proANP) to detect subclinical left ventricular hypertrophy (LVH) or LVSD was questioned in the Framingham Offspring's Study, in which the areas under the receiver operator characteristics (ROC) curve were less than or equal to 0.75 for both assays. Despite setting cut-off values that can achieve high specificity to detect cardiac dysfunction based on age and gender, less than one third of subjects who had abnormal LVH or LVSD could be identified by natriuretic peptide screening. These suboptimal performance characteristics of natriuretic peptide screening were substantiated by a large Japanese health-screening program. The ability of plasma BNP levels to discriminate between patients who did and did not have LVH also was limited (area under the ROC curve, 0.59; sensitivity, 50%; specificity, 69%; positive predictive value, 18.9%; negative predictive value, 90.5%) [49].

Patients who have a family history of heart failure or cardiomyopathy

Genetic determinants of BNP expression have been established in large epidemiologic studies [50]. A family history of heart failure is present in 30% of patients who have a history of heart failure [51,52]. Furthermore, recent data also suggest that up to 5% of patients who have heart failure may have an asymptomatic first-degree relative who has cardiac dysfunction that is significant enough to warrant intervention [53,54]. Genetic screening using the candidate gene polymorphism approach is extremely preliminary in this population [55], although asymptomatic relatives of patients who have familial dilated cardiomyopathy have increased plasma levels of N-terminal atrial natriuretic peptide [56]. Female carriers of abnormal genes that are related to muscular dystrophies also have higher plasma natriuretic peptide levels [57]. Nevertheless, there are no published data to support the routine use of screening for genetic determinants of BNP or NT-proBNP.

Patients who have other at-risk conditions

Several other clinical conditions have been considered as possible indications for cardiac screening, including sepsis [58–60], chronic obstructive pulmonary diseases [61], pacemaker implantation [62,63], lone atrial fibrillation [64–67], progressive valvular heart diseases [68,69], rheumatoid arthritis [70], pulmonary hypertension [71–74], and preeclampsia [75–78]. Although some of these conditions may not require the demonstration of cardiac dysfunction to warrant therapeutic interventions, using a simple blood test may facilitate careful monitoring and early detection of cardiac compromise in these at-risk conditions. Natriuretic peptide studies have been limited to case-control comparisons, and no prospective validation.

Summary

Prevention is not a new concept, but preventing heart failure progression largely has been ignored because of the knowledge and treatment gaps between patients, general practitioners, and cardiologists. As we ponder the epidemic of heart failure and the burden of health care costs for this condition, ignorance should no longer be an excuse for not exploring the role of early detection. Achieving conceptual changes by guideline implementation is the first step, but identifying tools and clinical recommendations are mandatory for implementation. If defining an appropriate "cut-off" for consideration of cardiac dysfunction hinders the progress of cardiac screening, there should be a re-examination of why cardiac dysfunction (and not increasing biomarker indicators of myocardial distress) is the gold standard for cardiac screening. We should learn from our colleagues in oncology and infectious disease; routine population screening and early preventive interventions are more likely to achieve public health benefits than are salvage strategies of heart failure therapeutics. With that thought, natriuretic peptides are the likely forefront candidate to achieve this important assignment, even if we need to abandon the traditional concept of detecting LVSD.

References

[1] Hunt SA, Abraham WT, Chin MH, et al. ACC/AHA 2005 Guideline Update for the Diagnosis and Management of Chronic Heart Failure in the Adult: a report of the American College of Cardiology/American Heart Association Task Force on Practice Guidelines (Writing Committee to Update the 2001 Guidelines for the Evaluation and Management of Heart Failure): developed in collaboration with the American College of Chest Physicians and the International Society for Heart and Lung Transplantation: endorsed by the Heart Rhythm Society. Circulation 2005;112:e154–235.

[2] Wang TJ, Evans JC, Benjamin EJ, et al. Natural history of asymptomatic left ventricular systolic dysfunction in the community. Circulation 2003;108:977–82.

[3] Freitag MH, Vasan RS. Screening for left ventricular systolic dysfunction: the use of B-type natriuretic peptide. Heart Fail Monit 2003;4:38–44.

[4] Davis ME, Richards AM, Nicholls MG, et al. Introduction of metoprolol increases plasma B-type cardiac natriuretic peptides in mild, stable heart failure. Circulation 2006;113:977–85.

[5] Tang WH, Girod JP, Lee MJ, et al. Plasma B-type natriuretic peptide levels in ambulatory patients with established chronic symptomatic systolic heart failure. Circulation 2003;108:2964–6.

[6] Ogawa T, Linz W, Stevenson M, et al. Evidence for load-dependent and load-independent determinants of cardiac natriuretic peptide production. Circulation 1996;93:2059–67.

[7] Wang TJ, Larson MG, Levy D, et al. Impact of age and sex on plasma natriuretic peptide levels in healthy adults. Am J Cardiol 2002;90:254–8.

[8] Redfield MM, Rodeheffer RJ, Jacobsen SJ, et al. Plasma brain natriuretic peptide concentration: impact of age and gender. J Am Coll Cardiol 2002; 40:976–82.

[9] Raymond I, Groenning BA, Hildebrandt PR, et al. The influence of age, sex and other variables on the plasma level of N-terminal pro brain natriuretic peptide in a large sample of the general population. Heart 2003;89:745–51.

[10] Tang WH, Philip K, Hazen SL, et al. Comparative sensitivities between different plasma B-type natriuretic peptide assays in patients with minimally symptomatic heart failure. Clin Cornerstone 2005; 7(Suppl 1):S18–24.

[11] Nielsen OW, McDonagh TA, Robb SD, et al. Retrospective analysis of the cost-effectiveness of using plasma brain natriuretic peptide in screening for left ventricular systolic dysfunction in the general population. J Am Coll Cardiol 2003;41(1): 113–20.

[12] Heidenreich PA, Gubens MA, Fonarow GC, et al. Cost-effectiveness of screening with B-type natriuretic peptide to identify patients with reduced left ventricular ejection fraction. J Am Coll Cardiol 2004;43(6):1019–26.

[13] McDonagh TA, Robb SD, Murdoch DR, et al. Biochemical detection of left-ventricular systolic dysfunction. Lancet 1998;351:9–13.

[14] McDonagh TA, Cunningham AD, Morrison CE, et al. Left ventricular dysfunction, natriuretic peptides, and mortality in an urban population. Heart 2001;86:21–6.

[15] McDonagh TA, Holmer S, Raymond I, et al. NT-proBNP and the diagnosis of heart failure: a pooled analysis of three European epidemiological studies. Eur J Heart Fail 2004;6:269–73.

[16] Bibbins-Domingo K, Ansari M, Schiller NB, et al. B-type natriuretic peptide and ischemia in patients with stable coronary disease: data from the Heart and Soul study. Circulation 2003;108(24): 2987–92.

[17] Silver MA, Pisano C. High incidence of elevated B-type natriuretic peptide levels and risk factors for heart failure in an unselected at-risk population (stage A): implications for heart failure screening programs. Congest Heart Fail 2003;9:127–32.

[18] Nakamura M, Endo H, Nasu M, et al. Value of plasma B type natriuretic peptide measurement for heart disease screening in a Japanese population. Heart 2002;87:131–5.

[19] Ng LL, Loke IW, Davies JE, et al. Community screening for left ventricular systolic dysfunction using plasma and urinary natriuretic peptides. J Am Coll Cardiol 2005;45:1043–50.

[20] Ng LL, Pathik B, Loke IW, et al. Myeloperoxidase and C-reactive protein augment the specificity of B-type natriuretic peptide in community screening for systolic heart failure. Am Heart J 2006;152(1): 94–101.

[21] Baker DW, Bahler RC, Finkelhor RS, et al. Screening for left ventricular systolic dysfunction among patients with risk factors for heart failure. Am Heart J 2003;146:736–40.

[22] Chatterjee K. All patients older than age 60 years should not undergo a B-type natriuretic peptide screening test. Am Heart Hosp J 2004;2:49–51.

[23] Richards AM, Nicholls MG, Yandle TG, et al. Neuroendocrine prediction of left ventricular function and heart failure after acute myocardial infarction. The Christchurch Cardioendocrine Research Group. Heart 1999;81:114–20.

[24] Richards AM, Nicholls MG, Yandle TG, et al. Plasma N-terminal pro-brain natriuretic peptide and adrenomedullin: new neurohormonal predictors of left ventricular function and prognosis after myocardial infarction. Circulation 1998;97: 1921–9.

[25] Richards AM, Nicholls MG, Espiner EA, et al. B-type natriuretic peptides and ejection fraction for prognosis after myocardial infarction. Circulation 2003;107:2786–92.

[26] Nichols GA, Gullion CM, Koro CE, et al. The incidence of congestive heart failure in type 2 diabetes: an update. Diabetes Care 2004;27:1879–84.

[27] Fang ZY, Prins JB, Marwick TH. Diabetic cardiomyopathy: evidence, mechanisms, and therapeutic implications. Endocr Rev 2004;25:543–67.

[28] Iribarren C, Karter AJ, Go AS, et al. Glycemic control and heart failure among adult patients with diabetes. Circulation 2001;103:2668–73.

[29] Bertoni AG, Hundley WG, Massing MW, et al. Heart failure prevalence, incidence, and mortality in the elderly with diabetes. Diabetes Care 2004;27: 699–703.

[30] Epshteyn V, Morrison K, Krishnaswamy P, et al. Utility of B-type natriuretic peptide (BNP) as a screen for left ventricular dysfunction in patients with diabetes. Diabetes Care 2003;26:2081–7.

[31] Magnusson M, Melander O, Israelsson B, et al. Elevated plasma levels of Nt-proBNP in patients with type 2 diabetes without overt cardiovascular disease. Diabetes Care 2004;27:1929–35.

[32] Fang ZY, Schull-Meade R, Leano R, et al. Screening for heart disease in diabetic subjects. Am Heart J 2005;149:349–54.

[33] Liew D, Schneider H, D'Agostino J, et al. Utility of B-type natriuretic peptide as a screen for left ventricular dysfunction in patients with diabetes: response to Epshteyn et al. Diabetes Care 2004;27:848 [author reply 848–9].

[34] Dawson A, Davies JI, Morris AD, et al. B-type natriuretic peptide is associated with both augmentation index and left ventricular mass in diabetic patients without heart failure. Am J Hypertens 2005;18:1586–91.

[35] Bhalla MA, Chiang A, Epshteyn VA, et al. Prognostic role of B-type natriuretic peptide levels in patients with type 2 diabetes mellitus. J Am Coll Cardiol 2004;44:1047–52.

[36] Wang TJ, Larson MG, Levy D, et al. Impact of obesity on plasma natriuretic peptide levels. Circulation 2004;109:594–600.

[37] Corboy JC, Walker RJ, Simmonds MB, et al. Plasma natriuretic peptides and cardiac volume during acute changes in intravascular volume in haemodialysis patients. Clin Sci (Lond) 1994;87:679–84.

[38] Tsutamoto T, Wada A, Sakai H, et al. Relationship between renal function and plasma brain natriuretic peptide in patients with heart failure. J Am Coll Cardiol 2006;47:582–6.

[39] Vickery S, Price CP, John RI, et al. B-type natriuretic peptide (BNP) and amino-terminal proBNP in patients with CKD: relationship to renal function and left ventricular hypertrophy. Am J Kidney Dis 2005;46:610–20.

[40] DeFilippi CR, Fink JC, Nass CM, et al. N-terminal pro-B-type natriuretic peptide for predicting coronary disease and left ventricular hypertrophy in asymptomatic CKD not requiring dialysis. Am J Kidney Dis 2005;46:35–44.

[41] Khan IA, Fink J, Nass C, et al. N-terminal pro-B-type natriuretic peptide and B-type natriuretic peptide for identifying coronary artery disease and left ventricular hypertrophy in ambulatory chronic kidney disease patients. Am J Cardiol 2006;97:1530–4.

[42] Nishikimi T, Futoo Y, Tamano K, et al. Plasma brain natriuretic peptide levels in chronic hemodialysis patients: influence of coronary artery disease. Am J Kidney Dis 2001;37:1201–8.

[43] Safley DM, Awad A, Sullivan RA, et al. Changes in B-type natriuretic peptide levels in hemodialysis and the effect of depressed left ventricular function. Adv Chronic Kidney Dis 2005;12:117–24.

[44] Mark PB, Stewart GA, Gansevoort RT, et al. Diagnostic potential of circulating natriuretic peptides in chronic kidney disease. Nephrol Dial Transplant 2006;21:402–10.

[45] Suzuki T, Hayashi D, Yamazaki T, et al. Elevated B-type natriuretic peptide levels after anthracycline administration. Am Heart J 1998;136:362–3.

[46] Conen D, Pfisterer M, Martina B. Substantial intra-individual variability of BNP concentrations in patients with hypertension. J Hum Hypertens 2006;20:387–91.

[47] Conen D, Zeller A, Pfisterer M, et al. Usefulness of B-type natriuretic peptide and C-reactive protein in predicting the presence or absence of left ventricular hypertrophy in patients with systemic hypertension. Am J Cardiol 2006;97:249–52.

[48] Dahlof B, Zanchetti A, Diez J, et al. Effects of losartan and atenolol on left ventricular mass and neurohormonal profile in patients with essential hypertension and left ventricular hypertrophy. J Hypertens 2002;20:1855–64.

[49] Nakamura M, Tanaka F, Yonezawa S, et al. The limited value of plasma B-type natriuretic peptide for screening for left ventricular hypertrophy among hypertensive patients. Am J Hypertens 2003;16:1025–9.

[50] Wang TJ, Larson MG, Levy D, et al. Heritability and genetic linkage of plasma natriuretic peptide levels. Circulation 2003;108:13–6.

[51] Goerss JB, Michels VV, Burnett J, et al. Frequency of familial dilated cardiomyopathy. Eur Heart J 1995;16(Suppl O):2–4.

[52] Michels VV, Moll PP, Miller FA, et al. The frequency of familial dilated cardiomyopathy in a series of patients with idiopathic dilated cardiomyopathy. N Engl J Med 1992;326:77–82.

[53] Matsumura Y, Elliott PM, Mahon NG, et al. Familial dilated cardiomyopathy: assessment of left ventricular systolic and diastolic function using Doppler tissue imaging in asymptomatic relatives with left ventricular enlargement. Heart 2006;92:405–6.

[54] Mahon NG, Murphy RT, MacRae CA, et al. Echocardiographic evaluation in asymptomatic relatives of patients with dilated cardiomyopathy reveals preclinical disease. Ann Intern Med 2005;143:108–15.

[55] Tiret L, Mallet C, Poirier O, et al. Lack of association between polymorphisms of eight candidate genes and idiopathic dilated cardiomyopathy: the CARDIGENE study. J Am Coll Cardiol 2000;35:29–35.

[56] Grzybowski J, Bilinska ZT, Janas J, et al. Plasma concentrations of N-terminal atrial natriuretic peptide are raised in asymptomatic relatives of dilated cardiomyopathy patients with left ventricular enlargement. Heart 2002;88:191–2.

[57] Adachi K, Kawai H, Saito M, et al. Plasma levels of brain natriuretic peptide as an index for evaluation of cardiac function in female gene carriers of Duchenne muscular dystrophy. Intern Med 1997;36:497–500.

[58] Bar SL, Swiggum E, Straatman L, et al. Nonheart failure-associated elevation of amino terminal pro-brain natriuretic peptide in the setting of sepsis. Can J Cardiol 2006;22:263–6.

[59] Hoffmann U, Brueckmann M, Bertsch T, et al. Increased plasma levels of NT-proANP and NT-proBNP as markers of cardiac dysfunction in septic patients. Clin Lab 2005;51:373–9.

[60] Brueckmann M, Huhle G, Lang S, et al. Prognostic value of plasma N-terminal pro-brain natriuretic peptide in patients with severe sepsis. Circulation 2005;112:527–34.

[61] Rutten FH, Moons KG, Cramer MJ, et al. Recognising heart failure in elderly patients with stable chronic obstructive pulmonary disease in primary care: cross sectional diagnostic study. BMJ 2005;331:1379.

[62] Thackray SD, Witte K, Ghosh J, et al. N-terminal brain natriuretic peptide as a screening tool for heart

[63] Gwechenberger M, Huelsmann M, Graf S, et al. Natriuretic peptides and the prevalence of congestive heart failure in patients with pacemakers. Eur J Clin Invest 2004;34:811–7.

[64] Nakamura M, Tanaka F, Sato K, et al. B-type natriuretic peptide testing for structural heart disease screening: a general population-based study. J Card Fail 2005;11:705–12.

[65] Lee SH, Jung JH, Choi SH, et al. Determinants of brain natriuretic peptide levels in patients with lone atrial fibrillation. Circ J 2006;70:100–4.

[66] Ellinor PT, Low AF, Patton KK, et al. Discordant atrial natriuretic peptide and brain natriuretic peptide levels in lone atrial fibrillation. J Am Coll Cardiol 2005;45:82–6.

[67] Arima M, Kanoh T, Kawano Y, et al. Plasma levels of brain natriuretic peptide increase in patients with idiopathic bilateral atrial dilatation. Cardiology 2002;97:12–7.

[68] Gerber IL, Legget ME, West TM, et al. Usefulness of serial measurement of N-terminal pro-brain natriuretic peptide plasma levels in asymptomatic patients with aortic stenosis to predict symptomatic deterioration. Am J Cardiol 2005; 95:898–901.

[69] Sutton TM, Stewart RA, Gerber IL, et al. Plasma natriuretic peptide levels increase with symptoms and severity of mitral regurgitation. J Am Coll Cardiol 2003;41:2280–7.

[70] Bhatia GS, Sosin MD, Patel JV, et al. Left ventricular systolic dysfunction in rheumatoid disease: an unrecognized burden? J Am Coll Cardiol 2006;47: 1169–74.

[71] Mueller T, Gegenhuber A, Dieplinger B, et al. Capability of B-type natriuretic peptide (BNP) and amino-terminal proBNP as indicators of cardiac structural disease in asymptomatic patients with systemic arterial hypertension. Clin Chem 2005;51: 2245–51.

[72] Mueller C, Laule-Kilian K, Frana B, et al. Use of B-type natriuretic peptide in the management of acute dyspnea in patients with pulmonary disease. Am Heart J 2006;151:471–7.

[73] Pruszczyk P. N-terminal pro-brain natriuretic peptide as an indicator of right ventricular dysfunction. J Card Fail 2005;11:S65–9.

[74] Leuchte HH, Holzapfel M, Baumgartner RA, et al. Clinical significance of brain natriuretic peptide in primary pulmonary hypertension. J Am Coll Cardiol 2004;43:764–70.

[75] Folk JJ, Lipari CW, Nosovitch JT, et al. Evaluating ventricular function with B-type natriuretic peptide in obstetric patients. J Reprod Med 2005; 50:147–54.

[76] Resnik JL, Hong C, Resnik R, et al. Evaluation of B-type natriuretic peptide (BNP) levels in normal and preeclamptic women. Am J Obstet Gynecol 2005;193:450–4.

[77] Kaaja RJ, Moore MP, Yandle TG, et al. Blood pressure and vasoactive hormones in mild preeclampsia and normal pregnancy. Hypertens Pregnancy 1999; 18:173–87.

[78] Furuhashi N, Kimura H, Nagae H, et al. Brain natriuretic peptide and atrial natriuretic peptide levels in normal pregnancy and preeclampsia. Gynecol Obstet Invest 1994;38:73–7.

[79] Vasan RS, Benjamin EJ, Larson MG, et al. Plasma natriuretic peptides for community screening for left ventricular hypertrophy and systolic dysfunction: the Framingham heart study. JAMA 2002; 288(10):1252–9.

[80] Costello-Boerrigter LC, Boerrigter G, Redfield MM, et al. Amino-terminal pro-B-type natriuretic peptide and B-type natriuretic peptide in the general community: determinants and detection of left ventricular dysfunction. J Am Coll Cardiol 2006;47(2): 345–53.

[81] Luchner A, Burnett JC Jr, Jougasaki M, et al. Evaluation of brain natriuretic peptide as marker of left ventricular dysfunction and hypertrophy in the population. J Hypertens 2000;18(8):1121–8.

[82] Landray MJ, Lehman R, Arnold I. Measuring brain natriuretic peptide in suspected left ventricular systolic dysfunction in general practice: cross-sectional study. BMJ 2000;320(7240):985–6.

[83] Smith H, Pickering RM, Struthers A, et al. Biochemical diagnosis of ventricular dysfunction in elderly patients in general practice: observational study. BMJ 2000;320(7239):906–8.

[84] Yamamoto K, Burnett JC Jr, Bermudez EA, et al. Clinical criteria and biochemical markers for the detection of systolic dysfunction. J Card Fail 2000;6(3): 194–200.

[85] Krishnaswamy P, Lubien E, Clopton P, et al. Utility of B-natriuretic peptide levels in identifying patients with left ventricular systolic or diastolic dysfunction. Am J Med 2001;111(4):274–9.

[86] Omland T, Aakvaag A, Vik-Mo H. Plasma cardiac natriuretic peptide determination as a screening test for the detection of patients with mild left ventricular impairment. Heart 1996;76(3):232–7.

[87] Ng LL, Loke I, Davies JE, et al. Identification of previously undiagnosed left ventricular systolic dysfunction: community screening using natriuretic peptides and electrocardiography. Eur J Heart Fail 2003;5(6):775–82.

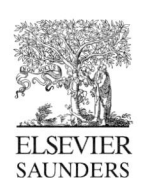

BNP for Clinical Monitoring of Heart Failure

Richard W. Troughton, MD, PhD, FRACP*,
A. Mark Richards, MD, PhD, DSc, FRACP
for the Christchurch Cardioendocrine Research Group

Christchurch School of Medicine and Health Sciences, Christchurch, New Zealand

Recent advances in treatment have led to increasing complexity in heart failure (HF) management [1–3]. Angiotensin-converting enzyme (ACE) inhibitors, angiotensin receptor blockers, and β-blockers are front-line therapy in systolic HF, with the addition of spironolactone in more symptomatic cases [1,3]. Additional vasodilator agents may be beneficial in selected patients [4]. Cardiac resynchronization and implantable cardioverter devices also improve survival in selected patients. Therefore, multiple decisions need to be made relating to treatment, including optimal dosing and timing of medication titration. In the setting of preserved systolic function there are greater challenges, mainly because of a lack of adequate evidence about effective therapy [1].

How best to optimize treatment for individual patients has become one of the major challenges of HF management [5]. Guidelines recommend optimizing proven therapies to doses achieved in landmark studies [1,3], but uptake of effective medications and titration to optimal dose falls well short of these targets in real-world populations [6,7]. One major reason is the lack of a validated objective guide to optimal drug dosing for individual patients [2]. As a result, some patients receive suboptimal treatment, whereas others may be overtreated, particularly with loop diuretics [8]. There is growing interest in developing more optimal strategies for monitoring HF, but lack of agreement as to the best method [5,9]. In most settings, clinical status is monitored primarily by gross indicators (eg, weight) and by physical examination. Despite the prognostic value of some physical findings [10], clinical signs do not reflect central hemodynamic disturbance or cardiac dysfunction accurately [11]. Symptom reporting by patients, functional testing by 6-minute walk or exercise testing, or echocardiography, to assess left ventricular (LV) filling pressures, are potential adjuncts to regular clinical assessment, but each has limitations (eg, lack of objectivity, logistic or resource constraints) and none is validated for routine monitoring [1,5].

Biomarkers play an increasing role in the management of cardiovascular diseases [12], and in many conditions, biochemical targets guide treatment (eg, low-density lipoprotein cholesterol in hyperlipidemia, plasma glucose in diabetes mellitus). Chronic HF is more heterogeneous with a broad array of etiologies and wide spectrum of clinical manifestation and risk; however, the B-type natriuretic peptides stand out as potential biomarkers for monitoring and optimizing HF therapy. They are validated diagnostic markers for HF and powerful markers of cardiac dysfunction and prognosis [13–19]. This article explores the evidence that serial monitoring with these peptides may provide more accurate risk stratification and guide more optimal treatment of HF.

B-type natriuretic peptides

The B-type natriuretic peptides are synthesized and secreted mainly from LV cardiomyocytes in response to increasing wall stress, particularly during diastole [20–23]. Significant atrial and right

---

* Corresponding author. Department of Medicine, Christchurch School of Medicine and Health Science, P.O. Box 4345, Christchurch, New Zealand.
  E-mail address: richard.troughton@cdhb.govt.nz (R.W. Troughton).

ventricular (RV) contributions are seen in advanced HF [24,25]. Cleavage of the precursor peptide (proBNP, amino acids 1–108) produces B-type natriuretic peptide (BNP) (77–108) and its corresponding amino-terminal component, NT-proBNP (1–76), which are secreted in a 1:1 ratio and can be detected in the peripheral circulation [22,26]. Plasma levels of these peptides correlate strongly with each other [15]. BNP is bioactive and has a shorter half-life as a result of clearance by neutral endopeptidase and natriuretic peptide C-type receptors; hence, levels are lower than for the more stable NT-proBNP by a factor of 5 to 10 [15]. Levels of both peptides increase with LV pressure or volume loading [22,27], and reflect the severity of LV dysfunction; they correlate inversely with LV ejection fraction (LVEF) and positively with increasing LV mass and indices of LV filling pressure [28].

Interindividual variation in B-type natriuretic peptide/NT–pro B-type natriuretic peptide levels

Plasma levels increase in HF in relation to the severity of symptomatic impairment and cardiac dysfunction [26,29]; however, there is wide interindividual variation in BNP and NT-proBNP levels in stable symptomatic HF because of many factors [24,30,31]. Levels of both are higher in women, lower in obese subjects, and increase with age, renal dysfunction, and atrial fibrillation [31–36]. Increased levels in renal dysfunction reflect reduced renal clearance because the transcardiac gradient—an indicator of secretion—is similar in patients who have impaired and normal renal function [31]. LV diastolic function, RV systolic function, and mitral regurgitation are important determinants of BNP levels; they presumably reflect left atrial and RV production in more advanced HF [24]. Up to 80% of interindividual variation in peptide levels is explained by LV systolic and diastolic function, RV dysfunction, renal function, age, and mitral regurgitation [24]. Hereditary factors may be responsible for a significant proportion of residual variation in BNP levels [37]. That BNP levels reflect multiple factors that relate to cardiac and end-organ dysfunction is a potential strength in monitoring the HF syndrome. BNP and NT-proBNP potentially act as markers of global status, rather than a single cardiac index (eg, left atrial pressure). A danger lies in an overly simplistic interpretation of BNP/NT-proBNP levels in isolation without considering factors that contribute to these levels [38].

A greater understanding of the factors that influence BNP and NT-proBNP levels has led to a more sophisticated approach to choosing cutpoint levels for accurate HF diagnosis, depending on age, gender, renal function, and other factors [39,40]. In the same way, this greater understanding should inform the choice of appropriate cutpoints or targets to guide treatment.

B-type natriuretic peptide/NT–pro B-type natriuretic peptide and hemodynamic indices

The relationship of B-type natriuretic peptides to cardiac hemodynamic indices is relevant to their potential use in guiding therapy. In stable patients with a range of cardiac abnormalities who underwent routine cardiac catheterization, clear positive correlations were demonstrated for BNP and NT-proBNP with indices of LV filling pressure [27,31,41]. These relationships are more complex in acutely decompensated HF. Most studies show that improvements in LV filling pressure, cardiac output, and systemic vascular resistance are accompanied by significant decreases in BNP or NT-proBNP levels [42–44]. A decrease in peptide levels identifies patients who improve clinically during treatment [42–44]. In acute HF, hemodynamic indices and BNP or NT-proBNP do not correlate significantly at baseline or after treatment [42–44]; this likely reflects small cohort sizes, a narrow spectrum of hemodynamic indices in severely decompensated patients, and other factors (eg, renal impairment). In one study in which BNP was measured on multiple occasions during 48 to 72 hours of hemodynamically guided treatment, a significant correlation was found between the decrease in BNP and the decrease in pulmonary capillary wedge pressure (PCWP) in the subgroup of patients that responded to therapy [42]. A further decrease in BNP was seen in the subsequent 24 to 48 hours, despite the PCWP being stable during that time; this indicated a lag between hemodynamic changes and the trough in BNP secretion [42]. This delayed response was seen in other studies [43], and is consistent with the known constitutive secretion of BNP [45].

In a separate study of subjects who had advanced HF and received hemodynamically guided treatment, although concordant decreases were seen for mean PCWP and median BNP levels 12 and 36 hours after treatment, there were no significant relationships between changes in hemodynamic indices and BNP [46]. In part, this may reflect the point of care assay used, which could not quantify levels above 1300 pg/mL, and the severity of illness in this high-risk cohort [46].

Although the routine use of a pulmonary artery catheter to guide treatment of severe HF is no longer indicated, there may be a role for hemodynamically guided treatment in selected patients who have acute HF [47]. Serial monitoring of BNP and NT-proBNP may identify the response to aggressive therapy with vasoactive agents. Peptide levels do not estimate LV filling pressure precisely and do not obviate hemodynamic monitoring where this is indicated. In combination with clinical assessment [48], however, peptide levels may identify patients who are not responding to therapy and for whom invasive hemodynamic assessment may be helpful to define the severity of dysfunction and to plan further interventions [9,47].

The relationship of serial changes in BNP and NT-proBNP to changes in hemodynamic indices in ambulant subjects with compensated HF requires some clarification. There are limited data on this topic; however, the recent development of devices that measure or estimate left atrial pressure in ambulant subjects has provided some insight in this regard [49–51]. One study evaluated ambulant patients who had chronic HF with an implantable hemodynamic monitoring system that estimated pulmonary artery diastolic (ePAD) pressure from an RV catheter [51]. Patients had serial estimates of PAD with simultaneous NT-proBNP levels during a 10-month period of follow-up. Among the 19 patients who were studied, the baseline level of NT-proBNP varied widely; there was significant variation in serial NT-proBNP levels and hemodynamic indices during follow-up. Analysis of the group as a whole did not identify any significant relationships between NT-proBNP levels and estimated PAD or RV systolic pressure at any single time point; however, intrapatient correlations demonstrated significant positive correlations between NT-proBNP and estimated PAD by the device (Fig. 1). These findings suggest that in individual patients, variations in NT-proBNP levels are related strongly to changes in hemodynamic status [51].

Intraindividual variation in B-type natriuretic peptide and NT–pro B-type natriuretic peptide levels

For serial BNP or NT-proBNP levels to be used to monitor HF, the variation in peptide levels within individual patients and the clinical relevance of this variation need to be defined. Few studies have described the variability in repeated measurement [52,53], whereas multiple studies have reported the clinical value of repeated measurements [14,17,18,43,44,54–57].

Differences in serial peptide levels reflect measurement precision (analytic variability) as well as changes in secretion (biologic variability). The former is a function of specific assay and peptide characteristics [26,58], whereas the latter reflects the complex network of stimuli and counterregulatory mechanisms that control peptide secretion [59].

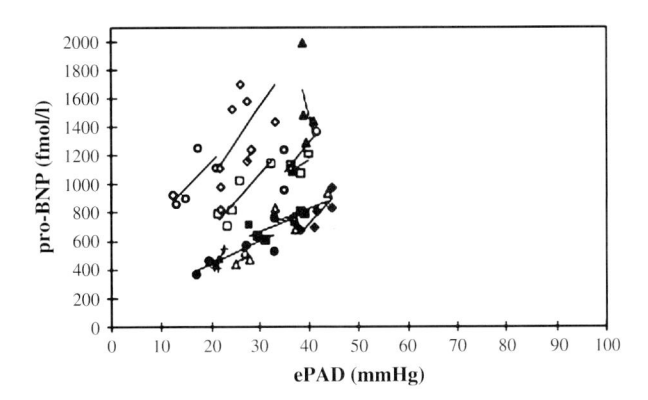

Fig. 1. Intrapatient correlations between serial measurements of NT-proBNP and the 24-hour median of estimated pulmonary artery pressure (ePAD; $P = 001$) in 13 patients who had chronic severe heart failure. Regression lines are drawn for serial measurements of each patient. (*Adapted from* Braunschweig F, Fahrleitner-Pammer A, Mangiavacchi M, et al. Correlation between serial measurements of N-terminal pro brain natriuretic peptide and ambulatory cardiac filling pressures in outpatients with chronic heart failure. Eur J Heart Fail 2006;[epub ahead of print]; with permission.)

Two recent studies assessed the variability of serial BNP and NT-proBNP levels in normal subjects and subjects who had clinically stable HF. Wu and colleagues [53] measured peptide levels in eight normal subjects (three men, five women) from four plasma samples that were taken at 2-week intervals. They demonstrated intraindividual coefficients of variation (CVs) of 33% for NT-proBNP and of 48% to 56% for BNP, depending on the assay used. They calculated that the smallest percent change in serial results that would be significantly different (with 95% confidence) from the combined analytic and biologic variation was 92% for NT-proBNP and 129% to 168% for BNP. As expected, this variability was lower for assays with lower analytic CVs—in this case 1.6% for NT-proBNP and between 1.8% and 16% for BNP, depending on the assay.

Bruins and colleagues [52] addressed the same question in 43 subjects who had stable HF, by measuring serial samples that were taken under standardized conditions within 1 day, on consecutive days, and weekly over 6 consecutive weeks. Median baseline levels were 134 pg/mL (interquartile range, 0–1640 pg/mL) for BNP and 570 pg/mL (17–5408 pg/mL) for NT-proBNP. They reported total CVs (including analytic CVs of 3% for NT-proBNP and of 8.4% for BNP) for within day, day-to-day, and week-to-week samples of 12%, 27%, and 41%, respectively, for BNP and 9%, 20%, and 35%, respectively, for NT-proBNP. Corresponding minimum percent change values for within day, day-to-day, and week-to-week samples were 32%, 74%, and 113%, respectively, for BNP and 25%, 55%, and 98%, respectively, for NT-proBNP.

In the authors' normal subjects (n = 8), they found CVs of 38% for BNP and 46% for NT-proBNP and corresponding significant serial change values (SSCV) of approximately 100% during serial testing at a 2-week interval under careful experimental conditions, including regulated diet and posture [60]. In reality, this reflected small absolute changes (± 9.3 pg/mL for BNP and ± 13 pg/mL for NT-proBNP) against a background of low mean peptide levels (8.9 pg/mL for BNP, 11 pg/mL NT-proBNP) that are not relevant to HF. In eight patients who had stable systolic HF under similar experimental conditions [61], CVs for samples that were taken 6 weeks apart were 10% for NT-proBNP, with an SSCV of approximately 30%, or 160 pg/mL against a background mean level of 550 pg/mL (Fig. 2). In 10 stable ambulant subjects who had HF who participated in a clinical trial of treatment that was guided by NT-proBNP levels [62], the CVs and SSCV for serial NT-proBNP measurements that were taken over 18-months were 38% and 105%, respectively. Applied in less stable patients from this cohort with higher peptide levels (>2000 pg/mL), this degree of variation represents a change of only 30%.

These findings in normal subjects and subjects who have stable HF indicate considerable variability in serial assay results that are due, in small part, to measurement imprecision, but mainly to biologic variation. The real question is, what causes this degree of biologic variability and what impact does this have on the clinical value of serial measurements? If serial BNP and NT-proBNP are to be understood within a framework of random variation around a homeostatic setpoint, the degree of variation described could make serial measurement meaningless, as inferred by previous investigators [52,53]. It seems likely that this view is overly simplistic and that the variation actually reflects clinically relevant alterations in peptide secretion that are due to active physiologic processes [58,59]. The secretion of BNP and NT-proBNP, although stimulated primarily by hemodynamic load, is under complex control and is modulated by multiple neurohormonal and immunologic factors, including angiotensin II, endothelin, and norepinephrine as well as by processes like ischemia [59]. These factors are highly dynamic and also contribute to cardiac remodeling and end-organ dysfunction in HF.

With regard to hemodynamic loading, monitoring with implantable hemodynamic devices has shown significant daily variation in indices of LV filling pressure, particularly in the setting of ischemia [50]. As described, these devices also demonstrate that serial NT-proBNP levels correlate strongly with indices of filling pressure [51]. These findings suggest that the biologic variation in BNP levels in patients who have apparently stable HF is not random, but instead reflects clinically relevant physiologic processes.

Clerico and colleagues [59] suggested that all variation in BNP or NT-proBNP that is more than three times the analytic imprecision of the assay in use (ie, more than three times the standard deviation of assay variability) should be regarded as clinically significant. In this context, immunoassays with the best imprecision (5% in some cases) will allow detection of smaller changes in BNP concentrations that may be clinically relevant [53,58,59].

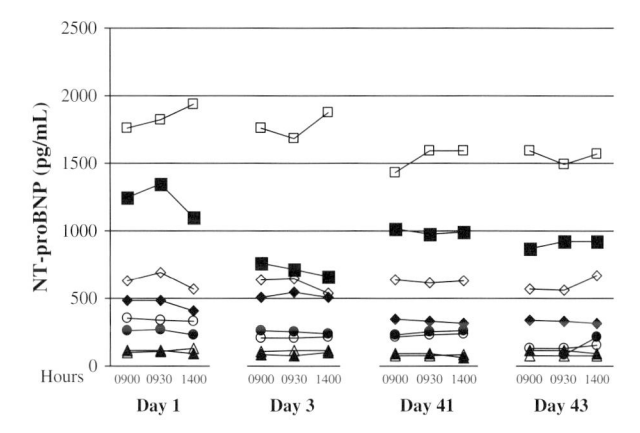

Fig. 2. Serial measurements of NT-proBNP in eight control subjects who had systolic heart failure who underwent blood sampling on four days over a 6-week period as part of an experimental protocol. Intraindividual coefficients of variation for serial NT-proBNP levels were 15% and 25% for samples taken 2 and 42 days apart, respectively. Significant serial change values were 232 pg/mL and 390 pg/mL, respectively, on a mean background level of 543 pg/mL.

Further studies are needed to better understand the basis for the biologic variation in BNP levels and its relationship to clinical status and outcomes; however, multiple studies have demonstrated the clinical value of serial testing.

Serial monitoring of B-type natriuretic peptides: incremental value for risk stratification

A large number of studies demonstrated the consistent finding that a single measurement of B-type natriuretic peptide is a powerful prognostic marker in HF. Typically, it predicts mortality and rehospitalization independently of LVEF, symptomatic class, age, and other key determinants of survival [13,16,54,55].

Recent studies demonstrated that serial measurements of BNP or NT-proBNP provide independent prognostic information that is incremental to single baseline values [14,43,63,64]. In the hospital setting, small cohort studies demonstrate that the highest rates of 30-day mortality and rehospitalization are found in patients in whom BNP or NT-proBNP levels increase, despite active treatment [14,63]. Although BNP or NT-proBNP levels at admission are useful for the accurate diagnosis and early management of HF [19,65,66], predischarge peptide levels seem to provide the greatest prognostic information regarding subsequent risk [16,63,67]. Whether routine predischarge testing alters management or outcomes is uncertain, but is being tested [68].

In the outpatient setting, Maeda and colleagues [17] measured BNP levels at baseline and 3 months after optimization of therapy in 102 patients who were hospitalized recently with severe (New York Heart Association [NYHA] III–IV) HF. Although BNP levels decreased after therapy was optimized, 3-month BNP levels remained the strongest independent predictor of the 26 deaths that occurred in subsequent follow-up. More recently, in the neurohormonal substudy of the Valsartan Heart Failure Trial, changes in BNP and norepinephrine levels during follow-up independently predicted survival in 4300 patients. Baseline BNP levels predicted subsequent mortality and hospitalization. Highest event rates occurred in patients with the greatest increase in BNP levels from baseline to 4 and 12 months, regardless of treatment group [55].

In considering serial measurement of BNP or NT-proBNP in HF, the most recent level seems to reflect the distance from decompensation, but more importantly is a powerful predictor of subsequent prognosis [63,69].

Serial measurement of NT-proBNP following acute coronary syndrome predicts recurrent myocardial ischemia, and persistent elevation in BNP after myocardial infarction predicts subsequent LV remodeling and scar formation [21,56,70–73].

Changes in B-type natriuretic peptide/NT–pro B-type natriuretic peptide in response to treatment

The response of these peptides to changes in treatment has been documented in a variety of studies of proven HF medications [13,74–76].

BNP or NT-proBNP levels decrease following institution of diuretic and vasodilator therapy [57,75], whereas withdrawal of diuretics is associated with an increase in peptide levels [77]. ACE inhibitors and angiotensin receptor blockers cause a decrease in natriuretic peptide levels [13,45,75].

The response to β-blockers is more complex. Introduction of metoprolol in stable mild HF is associated with an initial increase in BNP and NT-proBNP levels that reflects changes in secretion and clearance and is not associated with clinical decompensation [61,78]. Longer-term, BNP and NT-proBNP levels seem to decrease, possibly paralleling changes in LV remodeling [79,80]. The response to carvedilol and other vasodilator β-blockers, which may cause an initial decrease in BNP levels, seem to differ from that of metoprolol [74,81].

Prediction of response to therapy

Multiple studies have shown that BNP or NT-proBNP levels identify the subjects who have HF who are at the highest risk for adverse events during treatment and follow-up [13,54,55,76,82].

In the Australia–New Zealand Heart Failure Trial of carvedilol, 415 patients who had ischemic cardiomyopathy and LVEFs of less than 45% underwent blood sampling before treatment with placebo or carvedilol in addition to background therapy with ACE inhibitors and loop diuretics. The overall finding was a reduction in the composite end point of death and hospital admission. Prerandomization BNP and NT-proBNP predicted outcome, irrespective of treatment group [76]. In addition, both peptides seemed to predict a beneficial response to carvedilol, with the greatest benefit from carvedilol seen in patients who had peptide levels that were greater than the median [76,82]. Data from the Carvedilol Prospective Randomised Cumulative Survival Study in severe HF indicated a similar trend toward greater absolute benefit from carvedilol in the subgroup of patients that had the highest NT-proBNP concentrations [83].

Therapy guided by B-type natriuretic peptide or NT–pro B-type natriuretic peptide levels

Given that BNP/NT-proBNP levels in HF reflect the severity of cardiac dysfunction, identify the patients at highest risk, but decrease in response to effective therapy, it is possible that treatment that is targeted to decrease levels of these peptides toward the normal range could result in improved outcomes.

The effect of titrating treatment to decrease BNP levels has been studied in three randomized studies, of which two have been published. In the first, Murdoch and colleagues [75] demonstrated that titration of ACE inhibitor and diuretic doses that were tailored to decrease BNP resulted in significant reductions in BNP levels compared with standardized empiric treatment with these agents.

In a separate study, the authors studied 69 patients who had a history of decompensated HF, current NYHA class II–IV symptoms, and LV systolic dysfunction (LVEF < 40%) [57]. Subjects were randomized to have therapy adjusted according to a preset algorithm that was based solely on clinical status or according to serial plasma levels of NT-proBNP. In the "clinical" group, changes in drug treatment were dictated by clinical findings according to a formalized clinical score that was based on Framingham criteria for diagnosis of decompensated HF. In the hormone-guided group, treatment was titrated to achieve an NT-proBNP level of less than 200 pmol/L (approximately 1700 ng/L). Levels above this target triggered increases in therapy, even when the clinical score threshold was not exceeded (ie, even when there was no clinical evidence of decompensation or volume overload). If clinical or NT-proBNP targets were not met, dosages of loop diuretics, ACE inhibitors, spironolactone, long-acting nitrates, and other vasodilators were increased according to a predetermined sequence. At follow-up, NT-proBNP levels were reduced significantly below baseline in the hormone-guided group, but not in the clinical group. At a median of 9.5 months of follow-up, adverse clinical outcomes, including the primary end point of death, cardiovascular admission, or HF decompensation, were significantly lower in the hormone-guided group (Fig. 3). There were 19 adverse cardiovascular outcomes in 35 patients within the NT-proBNP–guided group, compared with 54 such events in the clinically managed patients ($P = .02$). Multivariate analysis allowing for minor intergroup differences in baseline features, including age, NYHA class, LVEF, baseline NT-proBNP level, and drug dosage, confirmed a more significant difference in clinical outcomes between groups than was seen with the unadjusted analysis ($P \leq .001$).

These findings were corroborated recently by a brief report of findings from a French multicenter

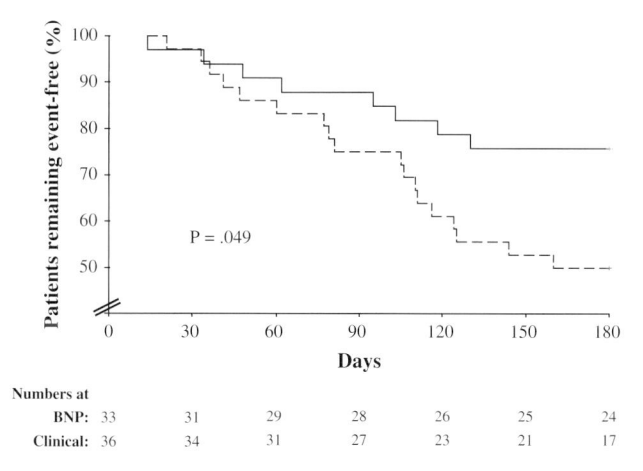

Fig. 3. Kaplan-Meier event curves for time to first heart failure event or death show a significant reduction in the events in that group whose treatment was adjusted according to serial measurements of plasma NT-proBNP. (*From* Troughton RW, Frampton CM, Yandle TG, et al. Treatment of heart failure guided by plasma aminoterminal brain natriuretic peptide (N-BNP) concentrations. Lancet 2000;355(9210):1128; with permission.)

study ("STARS-BNP") that was presented in abstract form at the American College of Cardiology Scientific Sessions [84]. Two hundred and twenty patients who had symptomatic HF (NYHA II–IV) and systolic impairment (LVEF <45%) were recruited in 21 hospitals and randomized to BNP-guided or clinically guided treatment. The two groups seemed to be matched for demographic and clinical characteristics other than LVEF, which was lower in the BNP-guided group (28 ± 7% versus 31.5 ± 8.6%; $P < .05$). Patients were followed for a median of 15 months; in this time there were significantly fewer events (death or admission to hospital for HF) in the BNP group than in the clinical group (25 versus 57; $P < .001$). HF events occurred in 15.6% of patients in the BNP group and 26.8% of patients in the clinical group ($P = .001$). The investigators concluded that in patients who had systolic HF and were treated according to standard guidelines, the use of BNP to guide medical therapy "reduced HF events and delayed time to first event compared with clinically guided treatment."

The concept of using NT-proBNP or BNP to guide treatment of HF is under scrutiny in larger studies [85,86], including a further New Zealand study: BNP-Assisted Treatment To LEssen Serial CARdiac REadmissions and Death ("BATTLE-SCARRED") [62]. In this study, patients with preserved or impaired ejection fraction are eligible. At 3 years, more than 2000 patients have been screened for participation in this trial. Of 511 eligible patients, 350 have been randomized to "usual care," intensively clinically guided therapy, or NT-proBNP–guided therapy. Patients have an average age of 77 years and more than half have ejection fractions of greater than 40%. Average NT-proBNP levels are fivefold the upper limit of normal and annual mortality is high at 22%. Prespecified secondary analyses for this study will include assessment of the efficacy of this treatment strategy in subjects who are younger or older than 75 years and in those who have preserved or impaired LV systolic function.

B-type natriuretic peptide/NT–pro B-type natriuretic peptide and monitoring in other settings

Short reports suggest that B-type natriuretic peptides may be useful in monitoring the response to cardiac resynchronization [87]. BNP and NT-proBNP levels correlate with symptoms in valvular heart disease [88,89], and potentially could be used in the monitoring of asymptomatic valvular disease to identify patients for whom intervention may be needed [90].

Summary

Recent evidence suggests that the B-type natriuretic peptides, BNP and NT-proBNP, may be useful for monitoring clinical status and guiding optimization of HF therapy. Plasma levels reflect the severity of symptoms and overall cardiac dysfunction. Serial BNP/NT-proBNP testing in the hospital or the community identifies the response to therapy and provides incremental risk stratification over a single baseline level. Follow-up levels reflect the distance from decompensation and provide a powerful estimate of the subsequent risk for HF events or death. These data could be used to identify high-risk patients for more intensive follow-up. The intra-individual variation in serial samples that are taken from stable patients seems to reflect subclinical changes in hemodynamic status and neurohormonal systems that regulate peptide secretion, and it does not seem to diminish the clinical usefulness of serial testing. BNP and NT-proBNP levels decrease with effective diuretic, vasodilator, and longer-term β-blocker therapy; however, levels after treatment optimization still predict adverse outcomes. Levels also may identify patients who are most likely to benefit from medical therapy. Recent studies suggest that titrating medical therapy to achieve BNP or NT-proBNP levels that are less than a target range may improve clinical outcomes compared with empiric strategies. These data suggest that serial BNP/NT-proBNP testing may be useful for monitoring response to therapy, determining the risk for future adverse events, and potentially for guiding optimal medical therapy.

References

[1] Hunt SA. ACC/AHA 2005 guideline update for the diagnosis and management of chronic heart failure in the adult: a report of the American College of Cardiology/American Heart Association Task Force on Practice Guidelines (Writing Committee to Update the 2001 Guidelines for the Evaluation and Management of Heart Failure). J Am Coll Cardiol 2005; 46(6):e1–82.

[2] Nicholls MG, Lainchbury JG, Richards AM, et al. Brain natriuretic peptide-guided therapy for heart failure. Ann Med 2001;33(6):422–7.

[3] Swedberg K, Cleland J, Dargie H, et al. Guidelines for the diagnosis and treatment of chronic heart failure: executive summary (update 2005): The Task Force for the Diagnosis and Treatment of Chronic Heart Failure of the European Society of Cardiology. Eur Heart J 2005;26(11):1115–40.

[4] Taylor AL, Ziesche S, Yancy C, et al. Combination of isosorbide dinitrate and hydralazine in blacks with heart failure. N Engl J Med 2004;351(20): 2049–57.

[5] Tang WH, Francis GS. The difficult task of evaluating how to monitor patients with heart failure. J Card Fail 2005;11(6):422–4.

[6] Hlatky MA. Underuse of evidence-based therapies. Circulation 2004;110(6):644–5.

[7] Stafford RS, Radley DC. The underutilization of cardiac medications of proven benefit, 1990 to 2002. J Am Coll Cardiol 2003;41(1):56–61.

[8] van Kraaij DJ, Jansen RW, Bouwels LH, et al. Furosemide withdrawal improves postprandial hypotension in elderly patients with heart failure and preserved left ventricular systolic function. Arch Intern Med 1999;159(14):1599–605.

[9] Nohria A, Mielniczuk LM, Stevenson LW. Evaluation and monitoring of patients with acute heart failure syndromes. Am J Cardiol 2005;96(6A): 32G–40G.

[10] Drazner MH, Rame JE, Stevenson LW, et al. Prognostic importance of elevated jugular venous pressure and a third heart sound in patients with heart failure. N Engl J Med 2001;345(8):574–81.

[11] Stevenson LW, Perloff JK. The limited reliability of physical signs for estimating hemodynamics in chronic heart failure. JAMA 1989;261(6):884–8.

[12] Mo VY, De Lemos JA. Individualizing therapy in acute coronary syndromes: using a multiple biomarker approach for diagnosis, risk stratification, and guidance of therapy. Curr Cardiol Rep 2004; 6(4):273–8.

[13] Anand IS, Fisher LD, Chiang YT, et al. Changes in brain natriuretic peptide and norepinephrine over time and mortality and morbidity in the Valsartan Heart Failure Trial (Val-HeFT). Circulation 2003; 107(9):1278–83.

[14] Bettencourt P, Azevedo A, Pimenta J, et al. N-terminal-pro-brain natriuretic peptide predicts outcome after hospital discharge in heart failure patients. Circulation 2004;110(15):2168–74.

[15] Lainchbury JG, Campbell E, Frampton CM, et al. Brain natriuretic peptide and N-terminal brain natriuretic peptide in the diagnosis of heart failure in patients with acute shortness of breath. J Am Coll Cardiol 2003;42(4):728–35.

[16] Logeart D, Thabut G, Jourdain P, et al. Predischarge B-type natriuretic peptide assay for identifying patients at high risk of re-admission after decompensated heart failure. J Am Coll Cardiol 2004;43(4):635–41.

[17] Maeda K, Tsutamoto T, Wada A, et al. High levels of plasma brain natriuretic peptide and interleukin-6 after optimized treatment for heart failure are independent risk factors for morbidity and mortality in patients with congestive heart failure. J Am Coll Cardiol 2000;36(5):1587–93.

[18] O'Brien RJ, Squire IB, Demme B, et al. Pre-discharge, but not admission, levels of NT-proBNP predict adverse prognosis following acute LVF. Eur J Heart Fail 2003;5(4):499–506.

[19] Maisel AS, Krishnaswamy P, Nowak RM, et al. Rapid measurement of B-type natriuretic peptide in the emergency diagnosis of heart failure. N Engl J Med 2002;347(3):161–7.

[20] Yasue H, Yoshimura M, Sumida H, et al. Localization and mechanism of secretion of B-type natriuretic peptide in comparison with those of A-type natriuretic peptide in normal subjects and patients with heart failure. Circulation 1994;90(1):195–203.

[21] Sumida H, Yasue H, Yoshimura M, et al. Comparison of secretion pattern between A-type and B-type natriuretic peptides in patients with old myocardial infarction. J Am Coll Cardiol 1995;25(5):1105–10.

[22] Mukoyama M, Nakao K, Hosoda K, et al. Brain natriuretic peptide as a novel cardiac hormone in humans. Evidence for an exquisite dual natriuretic peptide system, atrial natriuretic peptide and brain natriuretic peptide. J Clin Invest 1991;87(4): 1402–12.

[23] Iwanaga Y, Nishi I, Furuichi S, et al. B-type natriuretic peptide strongly reflects diastolic wall stress in patients with chronic heart failure: comparison between systolic and diastolic heart failure. J Am Coll Cardiol 2006;47(4):742–8.

[24] Troughton RW, Prior DL, Pereira JJ, et al. Plasma B-type natriuretic peptide levels in systolic heart failure: importance of left ventricular diastolic function and right ventricular systolic function. J Am Coll Cardiol 2004;43(3):416–22.

[25] Mariano-Goulart D, Eberle MC, Boudousq V, et al. Major increase in brain natriuretic peptide indicates right ventricular systolic dysfunction in patients with heart failure. Eur J Heart Fail 2003; 5(4):481–8.

[26] Hunt PJ, Yandle TG, Nicholls MG, et al. The amino-terminal portion of pro-brain natriuretic peptide (Pro-BNP) circulates in human plasma. Biochem Biophys Res Commun 1995;214(3):1175–83.

[27] Yoshimura M, Yasue H, Okumura K, et al. Different secretion patterns of atrial natriuretic peptide and brain natriuretic peptide in patients with congestive heart failure. Circulation 1993;87(2):464–9.

[28] Nishikimi T, Yoshihara F, Morimoto A, et al. Relationship between left ventricular geometry and natriuretic peptide levels in essential hypertension. Hypertension 1996;28(1):22–30.

[29] Lee SC, Stevens TL, Sandberg SM, et al. The potential of brain natriuretic peptide as a biomarker for New York Heart Association class during the outpatient treatment of heart failure. J Card Fail 2002; 8(3):149–54.

[30] Tang WH, Girod JP, Lee MJ, et al. Plasma B-type natriuretic peptide levels in ambulatory patients with established chronic symptomatic systolic heart failure. Circulation 2003;108(24):2964–6.

[31] Tsutamoto T, Wada A, Sakai H, et al. Relationship between renal function and plasma brain natriuretic peptide in patients with heart failure. J Am Coll Cardiol 2006;47(3):582–6.

[32] Redfield MM, Rodeheffer RJ, Jacobsen SJ, et al. Plasma brain natriuretic peptide concentration: impact of age and gender. J Am Coll Cardiol 2002; 40(5):976–82.

[33] Wang TJ, Larson MG, Levy D, et al. Impact of obesity on plasma natriuretic peptide levels. Circulation 2004;109(5):594–600.

[34] McCullough PA, Duc P, Omland T, et al. B-type natriuretic peptide and renal function in the diagnosis of heart failure: an analysis from the Breathing Not Properly Multinational Study. Am J Kidney Dis 2003;41(3):571–9.

[35] Luchner A, Hengstenberg C, Lowel H, et al. Effect of compensated renal dysfunction on approved heart failure markers: direct comparison of brain natriuretic peptide (BNP) and N-terminal pro-BNP. Hypertension 2005;46(1):118–23.

[36] Knudsen CW, Omland T, Clopton P, et al. Impact of atrial fibrillation on the diagnostic performance of B-type natriuretic peptide concentration in dyspneic patients: an analysis from the breathing not properly multinational study. J Am Coll Cardiol 2005;46(5): 838–44.

[37] Wang TJ, Larson MG, Levy D, et al. Heritability and genetic linkage of plasma natriuretic peptide levels. Circulation 2003;108(1):13–6.

[38] Nishikimi T, Matsuoka H. Routine measurement of natriuretic peptide to guide the diagnosis and management of chronic heart failure. Circulation 2004; 109(25):e325–6.

[39] Maisel AS, Clopton P, Krishnaswamy P, et al. Impact of age, race, and sex on the ability of B-type natriuretic peptide to aid in the emergency diagnosis of heart failure: results from the Breathing Not Properly (BNP) multinational study. Am Heart J 2004; 147(6):1078–84.

[40] Januzzi JL, van Kimmenade R, Lainchbury J, et al. NT-proBNP testing for diagnosis and short-term prognosis in acute destabilized heart failure: an international pooled analysis of 1256 patients: the International Collaborative of NT-proBNP Study. Eur Heart J 2006;27(3):330–7.

[41] Richards AM, Crozier IG, Yandle TG, et al. Brain natriuretic factor: regional plasma concentrations and correlations with haemodynamic state in cardiac disease. Br Heart J 1993;69(5):414–7.

[42] Kazanegra R, Cheng V, Garcia A, et al. A rapid test for B-type natriuretic peptide correlates with falling wedge pressures in patients treated for decompensated heart failure: a pilot study. J Card Fail 2001; 7(1):21–9.

[43] Johnson W, Omland T, Hall C, et al. Neurohormonal activation rapidly decreases after intravenous therapy with diuretics and vasodilators for class IV heart failure. J Am Coll Cardiol 2002; 39(10):1623–9.

[44] Knebel F, Schimke I, Pliet K, et al. NT-ProBNP in acute heart failure: correlation with invasively measured hemodynamic parameters during recompensation. J Card Fail 2005;11(5 Suppl):S38–41.

[45] Yoshimura M, Yasue H, Tanaka H, et al. Responses of plasma concentrations of A type natriuretic peptide and B type natriuretic peptide to alacepril, an

angiotensin-converting enzyme inhibitor, in patients with congestive heart failure. Br Heart J 1994;72(6): 528–33.

[46] O'Neill JO, Bott-Silverman CE, McRae AT III, et al. B-type natriuretic peptide levels are not a surrogate marker for invasive hemodynamics during management of patients with severe heart failure. Am Heart J 2005;149(2):363–9.

[47] Stevenson LW. Are hemodynamic goals viable in tailoring heart failure therapy? Hemodynamic goals are relevant. Circulation 2006;113(7):1020–7 [discussion 1033].

[48] Nohria A, Tsang SW, Fang JC, et al. Clinical assessment identifies hemodynamic profiles that predict outcomes in patients admitted with heart failure. J Am Coll Cardiol 2003;41(10):1797–804.

[49] Steinhaus D, Reynolds DW, Gadler F, et al. Implant experience with an implantable hemodynamic monitor for the management of symptomatic heart failure. Pacing Clin Electrophysiol 2005;28(8): 747–53.

[50] Ritzema-Carter JL, Smyth D, Troughton RW, et al. Images in cardiovascular medicine. Dynamic myocardial ischemia caused by circumflex artery stenosis detected by a new implantable left atrial pressure monitoring device. Circulation 2006;113(15):e705–6.

[51] Braunschweig F, Fahrleitner-Pammer A, Mangiavacchi M, et al. Correlation between serial measurements of N-terminal pro brain natriuretic peptide and ambulatory cardiac filling pressures in outpatients with chronic heart failure. Eur J Heart Fail 2006;19:[Epub ahead of print].

[52] Bruins S, Fokkema MR, Romer JW, et al. High intraindividual variation of B-type natriuretic peptide (BNP) and amino-terminal proBNP in patients with stable chronic heart failure. Clin Chem 2004; 50(11):2052–8.

[53] Wu AH, Smith A, Wieczorek S, et al. Biological variation for N-terminal pro- and B-type natriuretic peptides and implications for therapeutic monitoring of patients with congestive heart failure. Am J Cardiol 2003;92(5):628–31.

[54] Latini R, Masson S, Anand I, et al. The comparative prognostic value of plasma neurohormones at baseline in patients with heart failure enrolled in Val-HeFT. Eur Heart J 2004;25(4):292–9.

[55] Latini R, Masson S, Wong M, et al. Incremental prognostic value of changes in B-type natriuretic peptide in heart failure. Am J Med 2006;119(1):70. e23–30.

[56] Nagaya N, Goto Y, Nishikimi T, et al. Sustained elevation of plasma brain natriuretic peptide levels associated with progressive ventricular remodelling after acute myocardial infarction. Clin Sci (Lond) 1999;96(2):129–36.

[57] Troughton RW, Frampton CM, Yandle TG, et al. Treatment of heart failure guided by plasma aminoterminal brain natriuretic peptide (N-BNP) concentrations. Lancet 2000;355(9210):1126–30.

[58] Apple FS, Panteghini M, Ravkilde J, et al. Quality specifications for B-type natriuretic peptide assays. Clin Chem 2005;51(3):486–93.

[59] Clerico A, Zucchelli GC, Pilo A, et al. Clinical relevance of biological variation of B-type natriuretic peptide. Clin Chem 2005;51(5):925–6.

[60] Davis ME, Pemberton CJ, Yandle TG, et al. Urocortin-1 infusion in normal humans. J Clin Endocrinol Metab 2004;89(3):1402–9.

[61] Davis ME, Richards AM, Nicholls MG, et al. Introduction of metoprolol increases plasma B-type cardiac natriuretic peptides in mild, stable heart failure. Circulation 2006;113(7):977–85.

[62] Lainchbury JG, Troughton RW, Frampton CM, et al. NTproBNP-guided drug treatment for chronic heart failure: design and methods in the "BATTLESCARRED" trial. Eur J Heart Fail 2006;8(5):532–8.

[63] Cheng V, Kazanagra R, Garcia A, et al. A rapid bedside test for B-type peptide predicts treatment outcomes in patients admitted for decompensated heart failure: a pilot study. J Am Coll Cardiol 2001; 37(2):386–91.

[64] Bettencourt P, Ferreira S, Azevedo A, et al. Preliminary data on the potential usefulness of B-type natriuretic peptide levels in predicting outcome after hospital discharge in patients with heart failure. Am J Med 2002;113(3):215–9.

[65] Mueller C, Scholer A, Laule-Kilian K, et al. Use of B-type natriuretic peptide in the evaluation and management of acute dyspnea. N Engl J Med 2004;350(7):647–54.

[66] Davis M, Espiner E, Richards G, et al. Plasma brain natriuretic peptide in assessment of acute dyspnoea. Lancet 1994;343(8895):440–4.

[67] Bettencourt P, Frioes F, Azevedo A, et al. Prognostic information provided by serial measurements of brain natriuretic peptide in heart failure. Int J Cardiol 2004;93(1):45–8.

[68] Richards AM, Troughton R, Lainchbury J, et al. Guiding and monitoring of heart failure therapy with NT-ProBNP: concepts and clinical studies. J Card Fail 2005;11(5 Suppl):S34–7.

[69] Nishikimi T, Matsuoka H. Plasma brain natriuretic peptide levels indicate the distance from decompensated heart failure. Circulation 2004;109(25):e329–30.

[70] Vantrimpont P, Rouleau JL, Ciampi A, et al. Two-year time course and significance of neurohumoral activation in the Survival and Ventricular Enlargement (SAVE) Study. Eur Heart J 1998;19(10): 1552–63.

[71] Sabatine MS, Morrow DA, de Lemos JA, et al. Acute changes in circulating natriuretic peptide levels in relation to myocardial ischemia. J Am Coll Cardiol 2004;44(10):1988–95.

[72] Tsutamoto T, Wada A, Maeda K, et al. Effect of spironolactone on plasma brain natriuretic peptide and left ventricular remodeling in patients with congestive heart failure. J Am Coll Cardiol 2001;37(5):1228–33.

[73] Yan RT, White M, Yan AT, et al. Usefulness of temporal changes in neurohormones as markers of ventricular remodeling and prognosis in patients with left ventricular systolic dysfunction and heart failure receiving either candesartan or enalapril or both. Am J Cardiol 2005;96(5):698–704.

[74] Hartmann F, Packer M, Coats AJ, et al. NT-proBNP in severe chronic heart failure: rationale, design and preliminary results of the COPERNICUS NT-proBNP substudy. Eur J Heart Fail 2004;6(3):343–50.

[75] Murdoch DR, McDonagh TA, Byrne J, et al. Titration of vasodilator therapy in chronic heart failure according to plasma brain natriuretic peptide concentration: randomized comparison of the hemodynamic and neuroendocrine effects of tailored versus empirical therapy. Am Heart J 1999;138(6 Pt 1):1126–32.

[76] Richards AM, Doughty R, Nicholls MG, et al. Neurohumoral prediction of benefit from carvedilol in ischemic left ventricular dysfunction. Australia-New Zealand Heart Failure Group. Circulation 1999;99(6):786–92.

[77] Braunschweig F, Linde C, Eriksson MJ, et al. Continuous haemodynamic monitoring during withdrawal of diuretics in patients with congestive heart failure. Eur Heart J 2002;23(1):59–69.

[78] The Randomized Evaluation of Strategies for Left Ventricular Dysfunction Investigators. Effects of metoprolol CR in patients with ischemic and dilated cardiomyopathy: the randomized evaluation of strategies for left ventricular dysfunction pilot study. Circulation 2000;101(4):378–84.

[79] Stanek B, Frey B, Hulsmann M, et al. Prognostic evaluation of neurohumoral plasma levels before and during beta-blocker therapy in advanced left ventricular dysfunction. J Am Coll Cardiol 2001;38(2):436–42.

[80] Doughty RN, Whalley GA, Walsh HA, et al. Effects of carvedilol on left ventricular remodeling after acute myocardial infarction: the CAPRICORN Echo Substudy. Circulation 2004;109(2):201–6.

[81] Sanderson JE, Chan WW, Hung YT, et al. Effect of low dose beta blockers on atrial and ventricular (B type) natriuretic factor in heart failure: a double blind, randomised comparison of metoprolol and a third generation vasodilating beta blocker. Br Heart J 1995;74(5):502–7.

[82] Richards AM, Doughty R, Nicholls MG, et al. Plasma N-terminal pro-brain natriuretic peptide and adrenomedullin: prognostic utility and prediction of benefit from carvedilol in chronic ischemic left ventricular dysfunction. Australia-New Zealand Heart Failure Group. J Am Coll Cardiol 2001;37(7):1781–7.

[83] Hartmann F, Packer M, Coats AJ, et al. Prognostic impact of plasma N-terminal pro-brain natriuretic peptide in severe chronic congestive heart failure: a substudy of the Carvedilol Prospective Randomized Cumulative Survival (COPERNICUS) trial. Circulation 2004;110(13):1780–6.

[84] Jourdain P, Funck F, Gueffet P, et al. Benefits of BNP plasma levels for optimizing therapy: the systolic heart failure treatment supported by BNP multicenter randomized trial (STARS-BNP). J Am Coll Cardiol 2005;45(Suppl A):3A.

[85] Shah MR, Claise KA, Bowers MT, et al. Testing new targets of therapy in advanced heart failure: the design and rationale of the Strategies for Tailoring Advanced Heart Failure Regimens in the Outpatient Setting: BRain NatrIuretic Peptide Versus the Clinical CongesTion ScorE (STARBRITE) trial. Am Heart J 2005;150(5):893–8.

[86] Brunner-La Rocca HP, Buser PT, Schindler R, et al. Management of elderly patients with congestive heart failure–design of the Trial of Intensified versus standard Medical therapy in Elderly patients with Congestive Heart Failure (TIME-CHF). Am Heart J 2006;151(5):949–55.

[87] Sinha AM, Filzmaier K, Breithardt OA, et al. Usefulness of brain natriuretic peptide release as a surrogate marker of the efficacy of long-term cardiac resynchronization therapy in patients with heart failure. Am J Cardiol 2003;91(6):755–8.

[88] Gerber IL, Stewart RA, Legget ME, et al. Increased plasma natriuretic peptide levels reflect symptom onset in aortic stenosis. Circulation 2003;107(14):1884–90.

[89] Sutton TM, Stewart RA, Gerber IL, et al. Plasma natriuretic peptide levels increase with symptoms and severity of mitral regurgitation. J Am Coll Cardiol 2003;41(12):2280–7.

[90] Weber M, Hausen M, Arnold R, et al. The prognostic value of N-terminal pro B-type natriuretic peptide (NT-proBNP) for conservatively and surgically treated patients with aortic valve stenosis. Heart 2006;[Epub ahead of print].

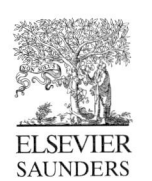

Natriuretic Peptides in Valvular Heart Diseases

Arti Choure, MD[a], W.H. Wilson Tang, MD[a], Roger M. Mills, MD[b],*

[a]Cleveland Clinic, Cleveland, OH, USA
[b]Scios, Inc., Fremont, CA, USA

Over the past decades, there have been dramatic changes in the approach to the diagnosis and management of valvular heart diseases. This improvement is attributable to extraordinary progress in the ability to quantify degrees of valvular abnormalities using echocardiography, the addition of potent new cardiovascular pharmaceutical agents to the pharmacopeia, breakthroughs in the design and manufacture of prosthetic heart valves, and dramatic advances in cardiac surgical techniques [1]. By relying on careful follow-up of echocardiographic measures over a range of time intervals, clinicians have also gained a better appreciation of the important differences between the effects of pressure overload and volume overload on cardiac structure and performance. The presence or absence of symptoms remains a crucial guide to the optimal timing of corrective surgery, however, as upheld by the latest guidelines [2].

Nevertheless, the natural history of valvular heart diseases is heterogeneous. Some patients may progress rapidly from an asymptomatic to a symptomatic state, whereas others may experience abrupt complications or sudden death [3]. Also, many patients do not report (or do not realize) the development of new or worsening symptoms immediately at their onset. Because echocardiography can be expensive, labor-intensive, and may require technical expertise in making accurate measurements, definitive decisions regarding the appropriate timing of corrective surgery can be challenging if echocardiography can only be performed in extended time periods (months to years). As a consequence, many patients who are referred for valve repair or replacement surgery have advanced myocardial dysfunction that may fail to improve or may even deteriorate following corrective surgery, leading to increased operative mortality and poor long-term survival. In contrast, premature intervention with valve surgery in asymptomatic patients may place them at risk for surgical and prosthetic valve-related complications, including infections and premature valve degeneration [4]. An easily measured, objective biomarker of early myocardial decompensation thus would be helpful in monitoring valvular disease progression.

Within a few years of the characterization of the natriuretic peptides, commercially available assays for B-type natriuretic peptide (BNP) and aminoterminal pro-BNP (NT-proBNP) were studied and validated as reliable aids in the clinical diagnosis of heart failure. These assays have proven particularly useful in the differentiation of cardiac and noncardiac dyspnea [5,6]. Overall, plasma natriuretic peptide levels correlate with New York Heart Association (NYHA) functional class and left ventricular (LV) function. Plasma BNP and NT-proBNP levels have also been studied as independent prognostic predictors in a wide range of cardiac and noncardiac conditions beyond acute heart failure syndromes [7–10]. Furthermore, BNP and NT-proBNP levels have been proposed as biomarkers for asymptomatic LV dysfunction [11,12].

Natriuretic peptide testing has been proposed as a marker of disease severity in valvular heart

* Corresponding author. Scios, Inc., 6500 Paseo Padre Parkway, Fremont, CA 94555.
   E-mail address: rmills@scius.jnj.com (R.M. Mills).

1551-7136/06/$ - see front matter © 2006 Elsevier Inc. All rights reserved.
doi:10.1016/j.hfc.2006.08.001

heartfailure.theclinics.com

diseases, especially in patients who have poor echocardiographic windows. This inexpensive blood test may provide the opportunity to monitor disease progression between echocardiographic testing intervals. Data regarding the use of these biomarkers in the setting of valvular heart diseases have been limited, however. This article reviews the published literature evaluating the role of natriuretic peptide levels in the evaluation and management of left-sided valvular heart diseases and attempts to synthesize the findings into pragmatic recommendations.

Natriuretic peptides in valvular heart diseases

In humans, the natriuretic peptide family consists of three main peptides: atrial natriuretic peptide (ANP), brain or B-type natriuretic peptide (BNP), and C-type natriuretic (CNP). All natriuretic peptides and their corresponding amino-terminal fragments circulate in blood and can be detected by various immunoassays. From a simplistic point of view, ANP is produced primarily in the cardiac atria and is released in response to increased atrial wall tension. In the normal heart, BNP, likewise, is synthesized primarily in the atria. As the myocardium fails or with the stimulus of ischemia, however, gene expression for natriuretic peptides are activated in the ventricular cardiomyocytes, and the left ventricle takes over as the predominate site for BNP production. This site-specific distinction is particularly interesting in interpreting plasma natriuretic peptide values in patients who have valvular heart diseases.

Cardiac hypertrophy in heart failure may lead to increased production of ANP and BNP. Their release into plasma is further stimulated by stretching of the failing atrial and ventricular myocardium and by elevated neurohormones, such as angiotensin II and endothelin-I. As "counter-regulatory" hormones, natriuretic peptides have been proposed to have diuretic, natriuretic, and vasodilator activities [13–15]. Furthermore, these endogenous hormones may also inhibit the growth of cardiac fibroblasts, retard collagen deposition and fibrosis, and limit the proliferative remodeling of the heart and the hypertrophic response to injury or ischemia [16]. Pathophysiologic processes that are active in various valvular heart diseases, however, may have different effects on natriuretic peptide expression, depending on the particular insult (pressure versus volume overload) and the site of injury (atrium versus ventricle) involved. For the purpose of discussion, this article focuses on isolated stenotic and regurgitant lesions of the two main valves in the left heart, mitral, and aortic valves.

Natriuretic peptides and mitral valve diseases

Mitral stenosis

Rheumatic mitral stenosis (MS) is still a prevalent disease in developing nations; the incidence of isolated mitral stenosis in developed countries has been falling. Normal mitral valve area is 4.0 to 5.0 cm^2, and symptoms may occur with reduction of the valve area to less than 2.5 cm^2, depending on heart rate and rhythm. Symptoms may result from increased left atrial pressure and reduced cardiac output that is caused by impaired left ventricular filling. Left ventricular performance, as determined by left ventricular ejection fraction (LVEF) often remains near normal in most patients, but high left atrial pressure and secondary pulmonary hypertension may lead to right ventricular dysfunction. The disease usually runs an inexorable, progressive course, with a predictable hemodynamic compromise caused by reduced preload.

Plasma BNP levels have been found to be higher in patients who have isolated rheumatic mitral stenosis compared with healthy subjects [17]. This was likely attributed to increased left atrial size and possibly right ventricular pressure loading, as extrapolated from the observations that plasma BNP levels can increase with the severity of right ventricular dysfunction in pulmonary hypertension [18]. In contrast to patients who have dilated cardiomyopathy, patients who have isolated MS have been shown to have a tighter correlation between pulmonary capillary wedge pressure (PCWP) and plasma ANP levels (but not with plasma BNP levels) [19]. These findings are suggestive of the primary pressure overload of the atrium with less impact on ventricular mechanics.

In general, natriuretic peptide levels directly correlate with left atrial dimensions, mean transmitral gradients, pulmonary artery wedge pressures, and NYHA class in patients who have MS, along with a weak but significant correlation with right ventricular dimensions [20–22]. Several studies focused on the ability of natriuretic peptides to track clinical changes following percutaneous balloon mitral valvuloplasty (PBMV) in patients who have severe MS [23–28]. These studies uniformly conclude that ANP is a measure of left atrial stretch and that ANP levels decline significantly after PBMV, indicating that reduction of ANP levels can be associated with successful PBMV.

The onset of atrial fibrillation (AF) in previously asymptomatic patients who have MS represents a risk for hemodynamic and cardioembolic complications. Because AF also signifies more advanced MS and potential surgical indication, elevated plasma natriuretic peptide levels follow the logic as a reliable biomarker for disease progression for MS. Among MS patients, those who have AF had significantly higher NT-proBNP levels as compared with those who have normal sinus rhythm [20]. Furthermore, plasma ANP and BNP levels decreased after PBMV for severe MS in the sinus rhythm group, but remained unchanged in the AF group [29,30]. Plasma ANP levels were not significantly affected by PBMV if MS patients were in AF [30]. Taken together, the observations from these observations suggest that in MS patients who have normal sinus rhythm, increasing natriuretic peptide levels might herald the onset of atrial fibrillation and thus might serve as a biomarker for timing of early intervention. With many limitations in the data, defining the use of natriuretic peptides, BNP, ANP, or NT-proBNP to help determine the timing for PBMV or to monitor the progression of MS requires further prospective studies.

Mitral regurgitation

Loss of mitral valve competence allows systolic regurgitation of blood from the left ventricle into the left atrium during systole. This results in the process of volume overload in the left ventricle, which receives the sum of right ventricular stroke output and the mitral regurgitant volume from the previous beat. Patients who have chronic mitral regurgitation (MR) may compensate for this volume overload by left atrial and LV dilatation and eccentric LV hypertrophy. As long as patients who have chronic MR have normal or decreased afterload, this increased preload may help to maintain LVEF [1]. The prolonged burden of volume overload eventually results in LV dysfunction, however, with an increase in peripheral resistance mediated by concomitant neurohormonal responses. MR may progress insidiously, causing left ventricular systolic dysfunction before the onset of symptoms [31]. The long-term prognosis may worsen once LV dysfunction occurs, with LVEF decreasing to less than 60% [32] or with end-systolic dimension exceeding 45 mm [33]. Quantitative assessment of the severity of MR, however, either measurement of regurgitant fraction or orifice area, is technically difficult. Furthermore, with a dilated left atrium serving as a pressure-volume sink, left ventricular performance as determined simply by LVEF may seem near normal even as LV dysfunction progresses [34,35]. These technical issues render optimal timing of surgery in patients who have MR difficult and have motivated several investigators to explore the usefulness of natriuretic peptide testing in improving the timing of interventions.

Plasma ANP, BNP, and NT-proBNP concentrations consistently increase with increasing severity of symptoms and severity of MR and left atrial dimensions [21,36–39]. Increased plasma BNP levels were also independently associated with the presence of functional MR in heart failure patients [21]. There were no correlations between any natriuretic peptide and LV dimensions or LVEF, however, which suggests that changes in ventricular physiology occur early in the course of disease, before echocardiographic evidence of increased LV dimensions. In multivariate analysis, adjusting for age and sex, the independent predictors of high plasma BNP levels were LV end-systolic volume index, LA volume, presence of symptoms, and AF [39].

There are limited data regarding changes in plasma natriuretic peptide levels with long-term outcomes and clinical status following corrective surgery in patients who have chronic MR. Asymptomatic patients who have severe MR and elevated plasma BNP levels have found to subsequently require surgery within 12 months because of development of symptoms [36]. Furthermore, asymptomatic chronic MR patients who have elevated plasma BNP levels but preserved LVEF may be at risk for experiencing postoperative cardiac dysfunction when compared with those who have lower plasma BNP levels [40]. These observational studies, however, were limited by lack of follow-up, small sample sizes, and subjective determination of symptomatic status. Regardless, elevated plasma BNP levels have been shown to be independently associated with higher mortality rates and with the combined end point of death or heart failure [39], similar to that seen in heart failure and myocardial infarction studies [8,40,41].

Focusing management decisions on either presently available echocardiographic markers or on symptoms alone has not led to optimal outcomes [42,43]. Based on the available data on natriuretic peptide testing, plasma BNP or

NT-proBNP levels have yet to provide additional information. There is, however, the potential for BNP or NT-proBNP to serve as an adjunctive biomarker to identify high-risk, asymptomatic patients who have chronic MR who need close monitoring for symptom development, and for those who have symptomatic MR and cardiac dysfunction who may be deemed too risky for surgical correction. Future large clinical studies on these issues are necessary before endorsing these indications.

Natriuretic peptides and aortic valve disease

Aortic stenosis

Aortic stenosis (AS) usually results from degeneration and calcification of the aortic trileaflet (in elderly patients) or bileaflet (in young patients) valve. The natural history of AS in adults consists of a prolonged latent period with low morbidity and mortality followed by the onset of symptoms, including angina, syncope, or heart failure. The development of symptoms marks a critical inflection point in the natural history of AS. The average survival after this point is on the order of 3 years. Indications for aortic valve replacement surgery include echocardiographic evidence of severe AS with corresponding symptoms or AS with an aortic valve area estimated at less than or equal to 1.2 cm^2 in asymptomatic patients undergoing concomitant open heart surgeries.

The timing of surgery in asymptomatic patients remains largely controversial. Current guidelines suggest that aortic valve surgery in asymptomatic patients may be recommended in the presence of LV systolic dysfunction, marked left ventricular hypertrophy (>15 mm) or valve area less than 0.6 cm^2 (class II recommendation). According to the latest ACC/AHA guidelines, no single clinical, hemodynamic, or echocardiographic measure has been adopted as a class I recommendation for surgical correction in AS patients in the absence of symptoms [1,2], because prophylactic surgery in asymptomatic patients would subject them to surgical risk and prosthetic valve-related complications that may outweigh their benefits [44,45].

The natural history of natriuretic peptide expression in valvular diseases has been best studied in the AS population. Because of the process of pressure overload leading to direct increase in wall stress, plasma levels of B-type natriuretic peptide are the highest of all isolated valvular disorders. Furthermore, plasma levels of natriuretic peptides correlated with left ventricular end-systolic wall stress as determined by invasive methods [46]. These findings parallel those reported in more symptomatic patient cohorts in whom plasma levels of natriuretic peptides correlated with severity of AS measured by transvalvular gradient and degree of left ventricular hypertrophy [47–49].

The logical extension of these findings is to determine if natriuretic peptide testing can help monitor patients who have "asymptomatic" AS. Gerber and colleagues studied the potential role of plasma natriuretic peptide levels as a marker for the onset of symptoms in 74 patients who had isolated AS and 100 healthy control subjects [50]. Patients underwent clinical assessment, echocardiography, and measurement of plasma BNP, NT-BNP, and ANP levels. The aortic valve area was smaller in symptomatic patients (n = 45; mean area, 0.71 ± 0.23) than in asymptomatic patients (n = 29), and plasma natriuretic peptide levels were higher in symptomatic patients than in asymptomatic patients. Also, the peptide levels increased with NYHA class, and these levels were significantly higher in patients who had NYHA class II symptoms compared with those who had NYHA class I. A progressive increase in natriuretic peptide levels was associated with decreasing valve area, but a sharp increase in plasma levels occurred as LVEF decreased to less than 50%. Furthermore in this study, less overlap of asymptomatic and symptomatic individuals were observed with natriuretic peptide levels when compared with standard echocardiographic measurements [51]. Natriuretic peptide levels hence can be potentially used to complement clinical and echocardiographic evaluations, and asymptomatic patients who have increasing levels can be followed more closely, keeping a low threshold for early surgery. Several retrospective studies now offer support for this hypothesis [52–57]. To date, however, no study has systematically and prospectively evaluated the role of natriuretic peptides in the management of asymptomatic patients.

As seen with MR and heart failure, plasma BNP levels in AS patients have been shown to independently predict cardiovascular mortality, even beyond clinical and echocardiographic evaluation [55]. Investigators studied BNP, NT-proBNP, and NT-proANP in 130 patients who had severe AS, 79 of whom required aortic valve surgery because of symptoms. Natriuretic peptides were found to increase with worsening

NYHA class and with decreasing LVEF. Furthermore, asymptomatic patients who developed symptoms during follow-up had higher entry plasma BNP and NT-proBNP levels than those remaining asymptomatic and had lower symptom-free survival. Plasma NT-BNP levels independently predicted symptom-free survival, and preoperative plasma NT-BNP independently predicted postoperative outcome with regard to survival, symptomatic status, and LV function. These findings have been confirmed by other similar reports [56].

Aortic regurgitation

Chronic aortic valve regurgitation (AR) produces left ventricular volume overload. In contrast to the retrograde flow into a compliant atrium in chronic MR, the large stroke volume in AR is ejected into the aorta, resulting in systolic hypertension and increased afterload. In the setting of combined pressure-volume overload, patients who have chronic AR often maintain a normal LVEF, recruitment of preload reserve, and compensatory LV hypertrophy. This well-compensated phase may last for decades. Patients decompensate when the imbalance between preload reserve, afterload excess, and hypertrophy results in LV dysfunction and reduced LVEF. No single hemodynamic measurement discriminates the boundary between normal LV systolic function and dysfunction adequately [1,2]. This means new biomarkers are needed to predict the onset of LV dysfunction before it becomes irreversible. Symptoms in aortic insufficiency may not occur until LV dysfunction is far advanced. Aortic valve replacement (AVR) should be performed before the onset of irreversible LV damage, even in asymptomatic patients [58,59]. The current guidelines recommend AVR in the presence of symptoms or in asymptomatic patients before LVEF decreases to less than 50% or end-systolic dimension exceeds 55 mm [1,2].

In 40 patients who had isolated chronic moderate to severe AR, plasma natriuretic peptide levels (BNP, NT-proBNP, and ANP) were evaluated as potential markers of LV dysfunction or symptomatic state [60]. All plasma natriuretic peptides were higher in symptomatic compared with asymptomatic patients and were higher in asymptomatic patients compared with normal control subjects. Correlations between natriuretic peptide levels and echocardiographic measures of cardiac structure and performance (including LV wall stress), however, were weak at best. The investigators thus suggested that increased LV volume alone may not be the major stimulus for increased natriuretic peptides and that the levels may increase in patients who have LV dysfunction even when LVEF is maintained. These findings were confirmed by a larger study by Ozkan and colleagues, who found increased plasma BNP levels that were significantly influenced by severity of AR [61]. As for the asymptomatic chronic AR patients, a small observational study found that the median serum BNP concentration in patients who had AR was nearly threefold higher than in normal control subjects and found a strong and significant correlation between plasma BNP and LV mass indices [62]. The underlying etiology of chronic AR may influence the detectable levels of BNP in the plasma, with bicuspid AR having near "normal" plasma BNP levels, likely because of the long duration available for remodeling adaptation for volume overload [63]. Again, there are no large prospective studies evaluating the role of natriuretic peptides in management of patients who have AR.

Summary

Increase in plasma levels of natriuretic peptides may reflect important pathophysiologic changes in the myocardium that can be related to progression of valvular heart disease. Plasma BNP and NT-proBNP levels have been proposed to predict symptomatic progression and to offer important prognostic information. To add more confusion, many patients may present with not just one but several valvular disorders (particularly in rheumatic heart diseases), and many may have confounding influences from failing myocardium. Better understanding of natriuretic peptide biology in the setting of valvular heart diseases is necessary before we can truly test the hypothesis that changes in plasma natriuretic peptide levels may occur before myocardial structural changes become evident. At present, therefore, the recently updated guidelines have yet to adopt natriuretic peptides as part of the diagnostic evaluation, partly because more data are needed to guide their use in this setting [2].

References

[1] Carabello BA, Crawford FA Jr. Valvular heart disease. N Engl J Med 1997;337:32–41.

[2] American College of Cardiology/American Heart Association Task Force on Practice Guidelines, Society of Cardiovascular Anesthesiologists, Society for Cardiovascular Angiography and Interventions, et al. ACC/AHA 2006 Guidelines for the management of patients with valvular heart disease: a report of the American College of Cardiology/American Heart Association Task Force on Practice Guidelines (writing committee to revise the 1988 Guidelines for the Management of Patients With Valvular Heart Disease): developed in collaboration with the Society of Cardiovascular Anesthesiologists: endorsed by the Society for Cardiovascular Angiography and Interventions and the Society of Thoracic Surgeons. Circulation 2006;114(5): e84–231.

[3] Pellikka PA, Nishimura RA, Bailey KR, et al. The natural history of adults with asymptomatic, hemodynamically significant aortic stenosis. J Am Coll Cardiol 1990;15:1012–7.

[4] Watanabe M, Murakami M, Furukawa H, et al. Is measurement of plasma brain natriuretic peptide levels a useful test to detect for surgical timing of valve disease? Int J Cardiol 2004;96:21–4.

[5] Maisel AS, Krishnaswamy P, Nowak RM, et al. Rapid measurement of B-type natriuretic peptide in the emergency diagnosis of heart failure. N Engl J Med 2002;347:161–7.

[6] Morrison LK, Harrison A, Krishnaswamy P, et al. Utility of a rapid B-natriuretic peptide assay in differentiating congestive heart failure from lung disease in patients presenting with dyspnea. J Am Coll Cardiol 2002;39:202–9.

[7] Nagaya N, Nishikimi T, Uematsu M, et al. Plasma brain natriuretic peptide as a prognostic indicator in patients with primary pulmonary hypertension. Circulation 2000;102:865–70.

[8] Richards AM, Nicholls MG, Espiner EA, et al. B-type natriuretic peptides and ejection fraction for prognosis after myocardial infarction. Circulation 2003;107:2786–92.

[9] Silvet H, Young-Xu Y, Walleigh D, et al. Brain natriuretic peptide is elevated in outpatients with atrial fibrillation. Am J Cardiol 2003;92:1124–7.

[10] Kucher N, Printzen G, Goldhaber SZ. Prognostic role of brain natriuretic peptide in acute pulmonary embolism. Circulation 2003;107:2545–7.

[11] Vasan RS, Benjamin EJ, Larson MG, et al. Plasma natriuretic peptides for community screening for left ventricular hypertrophy and systolic dysfunction: the Framingham heart study. JAMA 2002;288: 1252–9.

[12] Redfield MM, Rodeheffer RJ, Jacobsen SJ, et al. Plasma brain natriuretic peptide to detect preclinical ventricular systolic or diastolic dysfunction: a community-based study. Circulation 2004;109:3176–81.

[13] Levin ER, Gardner DG, Samson WK. Natriuretic peptides. N Engl J Med 1998;339:321–8.

[14] McKie PM, Burnett JC Jr. B-type natriuretic peptide as a biomarker beyond heart failure: speculations and opportunities. Mayo Clin Proc 2005;80: 1029–36.

[15] Yoshimura M, Yasue H, Morita E, et al. Hemodynamic, renal, and hormonal responses to brain natriuretic peptide infusion in patients with congestive heart failure. Circulation 1991;84:1581–8.

[16] Cao L, Gardner DG. Natriuretic peptides inhibit DNA synthesis in cardiac fibroblasts. Hypertension 1995;25:227–34.

[17] Golbasy Z, Ucar O, Yuksel AG, et al. Plasma brain natriuretic peptide levels in patients with rheumatic heart disease. Eur J Heart Fail 2004;6:757–60.

[18] Nagaya N, Nishikimi T, Okano Y, et al. Plasma brain natriuretic peptide levels increase in proportion to the extent of right ventricular dysfunction in pulmonary hypertension. J Am Coll Cardiol 1998;31:202–8.

[19] Yoshimura M, Yasue H, Okumura K, et al. Different secretion patterns of atrial natriuretic peptide and brain natriuretic peptide in patients with congestive heart failure. Circulation 1993;87:464–9.

[20] Arat-Ozkan A, Kaya A, Yigit Z, et al. Serum N-terminal pro-BNP levels correlate with symptoms and echocardiographic findings in patients with mitral stenosis. Echocardiography 2005;22:473–8.

[21] Davutoglu V, Celik A, Aksoy M, et al. Plasma NT-proBNP is a potential marker of disease severity and correlates with symptoms in patients with chronic rheumatic valve disease. Eur J Heart Fail 2005;7: 532–6.

[22] Iltumur K, Karabulut A, Yokus B, et al. N-terminal proBNP plasma levels correlate with severity of mitral stenosis. J Heart Valve Dis 2005;14:735–41.

[23] Waldman HM, Palacios IF, Block PC, et al. Responsiveness of plasma atrial natriuretic factor to short-term changes in left atrial hemodynamics after percutaneous balloon mitral valvuloplasty. J Am Coll Cardiol 1988;12:649–55.

[24] Hung JS, Fu M, Cherng WJ, et al. Rapid fall in elevated plasma atrial natriuretic peptide levels after successful catheter balloon valvuloplasty of mitral stenosis. Am Heart J 1989;117:381–5.

[25] Ishikura F, Nagata S, Hirata Y, et al. Rapid reduction of plasma atrial natriuretic peptide levels during percutaneous transvenous mitral commissurotomy in patients with mitral stenosis. Circulation 1989; 79:47–50.

[26] Nakamura M, Kawata Y, Yoshida H, et al. Relationship between plasma atrial and brain natriuretic peptide concentration and hemodynamic parameters during percutaneous transvenous mitral valvulotomy in patients with mitral stenosis. Am Heart J 1992;124:1283–8.

[27] Fujiwara H, Ishikura F, Nagata S, et al. Plasma atrial natriuretic peptide response to direct current cardioversion of atrial fibrillation in patients

[28] Ledoux S, Dussaule JC, Michel PL, et al. Acute and delayed hormonal changes in mitral stenosis treated by balloon valvulotomy. Am J Cardiol 1993;72: 932–8.
[29] Shang YP, Lai L, Chen J, et al. Effects of percutaneous balloon mitral valvuloplasty on plasma B-type natriuretic peptide in rheumatic mitral stenosis with and without atrial fibrillation. J Heart Valve Dis 2005;14:453–9.
[30] Razzolini R, Leoni L, Cafiero F, et al. Neurohormones in mitral stenosis before and after percutaneous balloon mitral valvotomy. J Heart Valve Dis 2002;11:185–90.
[31] Carabello BA, Nolan SP, McGuire LB. Assessment of preoperative left ventricular function in patients with mitral regurgitation: value of the end-systolic wall stress-end-systolic volume ratio. Circulation 1981;64:1212–7.
[32] Enriquez-Sarano M, Tajik AJ, Schaff HV, et al. Echocardiographic prediction of left ventricular function after correction of mitral regurgitation: results and clinical implications. J Am Coll Cardiol 1994;24:1536–43.
[33] Crawford MH, Souchek J, Oprian CA, et al. Determinants of survival and left ventricular performance after mitral valve replacement. Department of Veterans Affairs Cooperative Study on Valvular Heart Disease. Circulation 1990;81: 1173–81.
[34] Enriquez-Sarano M, Miller FA Jr, Hayes SN, et al. Effective mitral regurgitant orifice area: clinical use and pitfalls of the proximal isovelocity surface area method. J Am Coll Cardiol 1995;25:703–9.
[35] Corin WJ, Sutsch G, Murakami T, et al. Left ventricular function in chronic mitral regurgitation: preoperative and postoperative comparison. J Am Coll Cardiol 1995;25:113–21.
[36] Brookes CI, Kemp MW, Hooper J, et al. Plasma brain natriuretic peptide concentrations in patients with chronic mitral regurgitation. J Heart Valve Dis 1997;6:608–12.
[37] Sutton TM, Stewart RA, Gerber IL, et al. Plasma natriuretic peptide levels increase with symptoms and severity of mitral regurgitation. J Am Coll Cardiol 2003;41:2280–7.
[38] Mayer SA, De Lemos JA, Murphy SA, et al. Comparison of B-type natriuretic peptide levels in patients with heart failure with versus without mitral regurgitation. Am J Cardiol 2004;93:1002–6.
[39] Detaint D, Messika-Zeitoun D, Avierinos JF, et al. B-type natriuretic peptide in organic mitral regurgitation: determinants and impact on outcome. Circulation 2005;111:2391–7.
[40] Tang WH, Troughton RW, Agler DA, et al. B-type natriuretic peptide (BNP) predicts left ventricular response to surgery in patients with severe mitral regurgitation in asymptomatic patients with preserved left ventricular function [abstract]. J Am Coll Cardiol 2003;41(6, Suppl A):A509.
[41] Cheng V, Kazanagra R, Garcia A, et al. A rapid bedside test for B-type peptide predicts treatment outcomes in patients admitted for decompensated heart failure: a pilot study. J Am Coll Cardiol 2001;37:386–91.
[42] Enriquez-Sarano M, Tajik AJ, Schaff HV, et al. Echocardiographic prediction of survival after surgical correction of organic mitral regurgitation. Circulation 1994;90:830–7.
[43] Tribouilloy CM, Enriquez-Sarano M, Schaff HV, et al. Impact of preoperative symptoms on survival after surgical correction of organic mitral regurgitation: rationale for optimizing surgical indications. Circulation 1999;99:400–5.
[44] Carabello BA. Timing of valve replacement in aortic stenosis. Moving closer to perfection. Circulation 1997;95:2241–3.
[45] Pellikka PA, Nishimura RA, Bailey KR, et al. The natural history of adults with asymptomatic, hemodynamically significant aortic stenosis. J Am Coll Cardiol 1990;15:1012–7.
[46] Ikeda T, Matsuda K, Itoh H, et al. Plasma levels of brain and atrial natriuretic peptides elevate in proportion to left ventricular end-systolic wall stress in patients with aortic stenosis. Am Heart J 1997;133: 307–14.
[47] Prasad N, Bridges AB, Lang CC, et al. Brain natriuretic peptide concentrations in patients with aortic stenosis. Am Heart J 1997;133:477–9.
[48] Qi W, Mathisen P, Kjekshus J, et al. Natriuretic peptides in patients with aortic stenosis. Am Heart J 2001;142:725–32.
[49] Talwar S, Downie PF, Squire IB, et al. Plasma N-terminal pro BNP and cardiotrophin-1 are elevated in aortic stenosis. Eur J Heart Fail 2001;3:15–9.
[50] Gerber IL, Stewart RA, Legget ME, et al. Increased plasma natriuretic peptide levels reflect symptom onset in aortic stenosis. Circulation 2003;107:1884–90.
[51] Otto CM. Aortic stenosis—listen to the patient, look at the valve. N Engl J Med 2000;343:652–4.
[52] Lim P, Monin JL, Monchi M, et al. Predictors of outcome in patients with severe aortic stenosis and normal left ventricular function: role of B-type natriuretic peptide. Eur Heart J 2004;25:2048–53.
[53] Weber M, Arnold R, Rau M, et al. Relation of N-terminal pro-B-type natriuretic peptide to severity of valvular aortic stenosis. Am J Cardiol 2004;94: 740–5.
[54] Patel DN, Bailey SR. Role of BNP in patients with severe asymptomatic aortic stenosis. Eur Heart J 2004;25:1972–3.
[55] Bergler-Klein J, Klaar U, Heger M, et al. Natriuretic peptides predict symptom-free survival and postoperative outcome in severe aortic stenosis. Circulation 2004;109:2302–8.
[56] Nessmith MG, Fukuta H, Brucks S, et al. Usefulness of an elevated B-type natriuretic peptide in

predicting survival in patients with aortic stenosis treated without surgery. Am J Cardiol 2005;96: 1445–8.
[57] Gerber IL, Legget ME, West TM, et al. Usefulness of serial measurement of N-terminal pro-brain natriuretic peptide plasma levels in asymptomatic patients with aortic stenosis to predict symptomatic deterioration. Am J Cardiol 2005;95:898–901.
[58] Bonow RO, Lakatos E, Maron BJ, et al. Serial long-term assessment of asymptomatic patients with chronic aortic regurgitation and normal left ventricular systolic function. Circulation 1991;84: 1625–35.
[59] Carabello BA, Usher BW, Hendrix GH, et al. Predictors of outcome for aortic valve replacement in patients with aortic regurgitation and left ventricular dysfunction: a change in the measuring stick. J Am Coll Cardiol 1987;10:991–7.
[60] Gerber IL, Stewart RA, French JK, et al. Associations between plasma natriuretic peptide levels, symptoms, and left ventricular function in patients with chronic aortic regurgitation. Am J Cardiol 2003;92:755–8.
[61] Ozkan M, Baysan O, Erinc K, et al. Brain natriuretic peptide and the severity of aortic regurgitation: is there any correlation? J Int Med Res 2005;33:454–9.
[62] Eimer MJ, Ekery DL, Rigolin VH, et al. Elevated B-type natriuretic peptide in asymptomatic men with chronic aortic regurgitation and preserved left ventricular systolic function. Am J Cardiol 2004; 94:676–8.
[63] Sandhu R, Tang WH, Mills R, et al. Does the underlying etiology influence plasma B-type natriuretic peptide levels of patients with isolated chronic aortic regurgitation and preserved left ventricular function? [abstract]. J Card Fail 2004;10(4 Suppl):S52.

B-Type Natriuretic Peptides in Management of Acute Decompensated Heart Failure

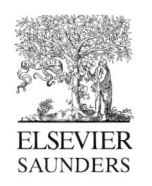

Clyde W. Yancy, MD

Baylor University Medical Center, Dallas, TX, USA

Acute decompensated heart failure (ADHF) has become a daunting clinical concern in the domain of heart failure. Whether defined as new onset symptomatic heart failure or a heart failure exacerbation in the setting of chronic heart failure, it is evident that ADHF must be considered as a unique and compelling disease entity. The most recent estimates suggest that heart failure as a primary discharge diagnosis accounts for over 1 million hospital discharges and over 6.5 million hospital days [1]. This care represents an enormous financial burden that is largely borne by Medicare. Of even greater concern are the prognostic implications of an episode of ADHF. The 6-month readmission rate is 50%, and the mortality rate at 60 to 90 days remains approximately 10%, with the 1-year risk of death approximately 30% [2,3]. When compared with well-treated chronic heart failure, the 1-year risk of death after an episode of ADHF is tripled. Whereas an impressive array of effective evidence-based strategies exist in the management of chronic heart failure, this is not true for ADHF. Recently, acute heart failure guidelines have been developed to assist practitioners, but these guidelines are proposed in the context of a dearth of clinical trial data demonstrating effective amelioration of hard clinical outcomes, especially rehospitalization and near- and intermediate-term mortality risk (Box 1) [2,4]. To date, no medical treatment strategy for ADHF has been proven to impact favorably the natural history of the disease.

The dilemma is that the pathophysiology of ADHF is not fully understood. Given the abrupt change in the natural history that follows an episode of ADHF, one can intuit that any of several circumstances may be operative: (1) a change in the ventricular substrate, that is, ventricular injury; (2) an act of commission, such as in a treatment option, that results in deleterious outcomes; (3) an act of omission, that is, a failure to address a critical risk factor or to introduce the correct therapies; or (4) faulty disease management after an episode of ADHF. Once an episode of ADHF is established, it is clear that hemodynamic derangements are responsible for symptoms, and correcting these derangements represents the only contemporary treatment objective in the management of ADHF. The hemodynamic alterations seen in ADHF are likely surrogates of the actual pathophysiologic derangements, and until those circumstances are better elucidated, the treatment of ADHF will remain problematic.

Current treatment schemes are based on an assessment of the absence or presence of congestion, low or normal cardiac output, and normal, low, or elevated systemic blood pressure. Data from the Acute Decompensated Heart Failure Registry (ADHERE) database clearly demonstrate that congestion is the overwhelming clinical scenario that heralds an episode of ADHF in the general community [5]. The Evaluation Study of Congestive Heart Failure and Pulmonary Artery Catheterization Effectiveness (ESCAPE) trial extends the profile to congestion and low output states in patients with advanced heart failure who present to tertiary medical centers with acute decompensation [6].

E-mail address: clydey@baylorhealth.edu

> **Box 1. Heart Failure Society of America practice guidelines for acute decompensated heart failure**
>
> *Evaluation and management of patients with ADHF: overall recommendations*
> - Patients admitted with ADHF and evidence of fluid overload should be treated initially with loop diuretics.
> - When congestion fails to improve in response to diuretic therapy, the following options should be considered:
>   Sodium and fluid restriction
>   Increased doses of loop diuretics
>   Continuous infusion of a loop diuretic
>   Addition of a second type of diuretic
>   Ultrafiltration
> - In the absence of symptomatic hypotension, intravenous nitroglycerin, sodium nitroprusside, or nesiritide may be considered as an addition to diuretic therapy for rapid improvement of congestive symptoms in patients with ADHF.
>
> *Evaluation and management of patients with ADHF: specific recommendations*
> - 12.15. In the absence of hypotension, intravenous nitroglycerin, sodium nitroprusside, or nesiritide may be considered as an addition to diuretic therapy for rapid improvement of congestive symptoms in patients admitted with ADHF. [Strength of evidence B.]
> - 12.16. Intravenous vasodilators (nitroglycerin or sodium nitroprusside) and diuretics are recommended for rapid relief in patients with acute pulmonary edema or severe hypertension.
> - 12.17. Intravenous vasodilators (sodium nitroprusside, nitroglycerin, or nesiritide) may be considered in patients with ADHF and advanced heart failure who have persistent severe heart failure despite aggressive treatment with diuretics and standard oral therapies. [Strength of evidence C.]
> - Intravenous inotropes (milrinone or dobutamine) may be considered to relieve symptoms and improve end-organ function in patients with advanced heart failure.
>
> *Modified from* Heart Failure Society of America. Executive Summary: HFSA 2006 comprehensive heart failure practice guideline. J Card Fail 2006:12;10–38; with permission.

Current therapies

Diuretics, mechanical volume removal, inotropes, and vasodilators represent currently available treatment options for ADHF. Background therapy should be consistent with evidence-based guidelines for chronic heart failure. Diuretic therapy is the mainstay of treatment for ADHF because removal of extracellular fluid volume leads to decongestion and prompt relief of symptoms. No clinical trials have been done to evaluate the effect of diuretic therapy on the natural history of ADHF. Registry data from ADHERE raise a concern that diuretic therapy for ADHF is not without risk. In an evaluation of more than 50,000 hospital admissions in the ADHERE study, the use of intravenous diuretics increased the risk of in-hospital mortality (odds ratio [OR], 1.29; 95% confidence interval [CI], 1.04–1.59) after adjusting for baseline covariates and treatment propensity [7]. It is well known that acute parenteral administration of loop diuretics results in an elevation in pulmonary artery pressures, an increase in systemic vascular resistance, and a reduction in the glomerular filtration rate [8,9]. Of greater concern is the well-described increase in neurohormonal activation associated with diuretic administration [10]. This response is seemingly counterproductive in the setting of an exacerbation of heart failure. Similarly, diuretic therapy given for chronic heart failure may be associated with a less good prognosis [11,12], and animal data suggest that structural changes in the renal tubule occur in the setting of chronic administration of high-dose loop diuretics

[13]. This effective and common treatment of ADHF may not be entirely benign.

Recent data testing the benefit of ultrafiltration are promising. The UNLOAD trial (Ultrafiltration versus IV Diuretics for Patients Hospitalized for Acute Decompensated Congestive Heart Failure) demonstrated that patients randomized to ultrafiltration instead of diuretic therapy for decompensated heart failure experienced a greater weight loss and volume removal, a similar improvement in the symptoms of dyspnea, and a provocative signal of reduction in near-term rehospitalization. These data were accrued early in the development of this treatment strategy, and the correct interface of mechanical volume removal with conventional therapy for ADHF has not yet been determined [14].

Inotropic therapy has been demonstrated consistently to lead to less good outcomes in the treatment of ADHF. When inodilator therapy, that is, milrinone, was compared with placebo in the OPTIME trial (Outcomes of a Prospective Trial of Intravenous Milrinone for Exacerbations of Chronic Heart Failure), more adverse clinical events occurred on active therapy than with placebo [15]. In the ESCAPE trial, the use of inotropic agents was associated with an increased risk of death (hazard ratio [HR], 1.75; 95% CI, 1.05–2.92) and death plus rehospitalization (HR, 2.12; 95% CI, 1.52–2.97) after adjustment for blood pressure and renal function [6]. Recently, a new class of inotropes, calcium sensitizers, has been investigated. The SURVIVE (Survival of Patients with Acute Heart Failure in Need of Intravenous Inotropic Support) trial specifically assessed the benefit of levosimendan. This trial found no significant differences between patients randomized to levosimendan versus dobutamine in the primary endpoint of all-cause mortality at 180 days (HR, 0.91; 95% CI, 0.74–1.13) or the secondary endpoints of all-cause mortality at 5 days (HR, 0.72; 95% CI, 0.44–1.16) or 31 days (HR, 0.85; 95% CI, 0.63–1.15) [16]. In the REVIVE-II (Randomized Evaluations of Levosimendan) trial, the secondary endpoint of 90-day mortality was greater, although not significantly, in patients randomized to levosimendan (15.1%) versus placebo (11.6%) [17]. These investigations revealed a sufficient signal of risk such that further development of these compounds is likely on hold. The use of inotropes in the setting of ADHF should be reserved for patients with frank or impending cardiogenic shock.

Vasodilator therapy is especially attractive as a treatment option for ADHF given that filling pressures are lowered, cardiac output is improved without increasing myocardial oxygen consumption, and blood pressure can be preserved. Again, there are no data to suggest a survival advantage or a benefit on rehospitalization after an episode of ADHF, but sufficient data exist to suggest that outcomes are better on vasodilator therapy than on inotropic therapy for ADHF [18]. The available vasodilators include nitroglycerin, nitroprusside, and B-type natriuretic peptide (ie, nesiritide). Nitroglycerin is a venodilator that also increases coronary artery blood flow and has an acute hemodynamic effect that is favorable. Intravenous nitroglycerin administered for ADHF is associated with acute symptom relief without a signal of apparent increase in risk; however, nitrate tolerance is well described and may occur early if the dose administered is elevated. Headache may make the therapy difficult to administer or titrate. No clinical trials to date have demonstrated a survival advantage associated with the use of nitroglycerin, but, similarly, there has been no evidence of risk associated with parenteral therapy with nitroglycerin. Nitroprusside is a balanced vasodilator that promotes arterial and venous vasodilation. For patients who have hemodynamic profiles in ADHF that are characterized by a low cardiac output and increased systemic vascular resistance, the administration of nitroprusside can lead to dramatic clinical improvement with marked increases in cardiac output and subsequent hemodynamic stability. These benefits are not long lasting because thiocyanide toxicity occurs and can be problematic, requiring acute intervention. The risk for thiocyanide toxicity is increased in the older patient, in the setting of chronic liver disease, and with chronic renal disease. Reflex tachycardia, profound hypotension, and activation of neurohormonal systems may also be associated with nitroglycerin and nitroprusside therapy [19].

Nesiritide: a therapeutic application of B-type natriuretic peptides

Nesiritide is a synthetic form of human B-type natriuretic peptide. It is synthesized using recombinant technology from *Escherichia coli* and is structurally identical to the endogenous hormone [20]. It has a ligand-receptor interaction with natriuretic peptide receptor-A which results in activation of guanylate cyclase and yields a subsequent intracellular increase in the second messenger cyclic guanosine monophosphate (cGMP). Among the properties exerted by the production of cGMP is a direct relaxant effect on human vascular tissue [20,21]. In healthy volunteers and individuals with heart failure, this effect of nesiritide produces a balanced vasodilation, significantly reducing mean arterial pressure, pulmonary capillary wedge pressure (PCWP), and right atrial pressure [22]. In an evaluation of 19 patients with severe heart failure, nesiritide produced a 48% reduction in mean PCWP and a 56% reduction in mean right atrial pressure (for both, $P < 0.01$ versus placebo) [23]. In another evaluation of 16 patients with ADHF, nesiritide produced a 17% reduction in mean arterial pressure ($P < .001$), a 41% reduction in PCWP ($P < .001$), and a 31% reduction in right atrial pressure ($P < .001$) versus placebo. This vasodilation produced an increase in the cardiac index and coronary blood flow [22]. In an evaluation of 10 patients undergoing heart catheterization, nesiritide increased coronary artery diameter by 15% ($P = .007$), coronary velocity by 14% ($P = .015$), and coronary blood flow by 35% ($P = .007$) while reducing coronary resistance by 23% ($P = .036$) versus placebo [24]. These changes occurred without a significant increase in heart rate, which is a crude marker of chronotropic activity and myocardial oxygen consumption.

Nesiritide differs from all other parenterally administered compounds in that it has at least a neutral if not potentially beneficial neurohormonal profile [25–27]. Nesiritide inhibits sympathetic stimulation centrally and in the periphery. Circulating levels of norepinephrine are diminished after administration of nesiritide [25]. In a randomized multicenter evaluation, nesiritide at a dose of 0.015 µg/kg/min improved several markers of heart rate variability, another marker of sympathetic activation. These data included standard deviation of the R-R intervals over 24 hours ($P = .001$), standard deviation of all 5-minute mean R-R intervals ($P = .02$), and the square root of mean squared differences of successive R-R intervals ($P = .01$) in patients with severely depressed heart rate variability at baseline [28]. This observation is consistent with an inhibition of the sympathetic nervous system and at least a partial correction of the sympathetic-parasympathetic balance. Data also demonstrate the potential of nesiritide to inhibit the renin-angiotensin-aldosterone system. The strongest signal appears to be in modulating aldosterone levels [25,27]. It is intriguing to acknowledge that aldosterone has emerged as an important marker of left ventricular remodeling with its greatest effect on left ventricular fibrosis. Major clinical trial data from the Randomized Aldactone Evaluation Study (RALES) [29] and Eplerenone Post-Acute Myocardial Infarction Heart Failure Efficacy and Survival Study (EPHESUS) [30] have confirmed the significant advantages of aldosterone antagonism in the setting of chronic heart failure or post myocardial infarction left ventricular dysfunction. In the setting of acute heart failure and chronic decompensated heart failure, nesiritide has been demonstrated to lower aldosterone levels [25,27,31]. Nesiritide also inhibits the endothelin system [32]. Endothelin-1 is a potent vasoconstrictor and growth promoter and generates cytokine activation, especially via its effects on transforming growth factor beta-1. In patients with decompensated heart failure, nesiritide (0.015 µg/kg/min) has been shown to lower endothelin-1 levels by 20% ($P < .001$) [32].

In healthy volunteers, nesiritide increases the glomerular filtration rate and produces a diuresis and natriuresis in a dose-dependent fashion [33–35]. In the kidney, it inhibits sodium resorption in the proximal and distal nephron, with its major effect occurring in the distal nephron [34]. Nesiritide also inhibits the tubuloglomerular feedback response that would typically occur in response to increased salt delivery in the distal tubule, preserving this natriuretic effect [36]. In patients with heart failure, the renal effects of nesiritide are less well established and may indeed be deleterious for undetermined reasons. In a small study, hospitalized patients with stable left ventricular dysfunction were randomized to nesiritide versus placebo. There was no incremental increase in natriuresis in the patients treated with nesiritide [37]. Several factors may be operative, including the intravascular volume status, concomitant medications, especially diuretics, and the underlying degree of comorbid renal insufficiency. Multiple small studies have shown nesiritide to have variable effects on renal blood flow, glomerular filtration rate, urinary sodium excretion, and water excretion [37,38]. No definitive statement can be made that nesiritide is renoprotective as it is currently administered.

Nesiritide as a therapeutic option for acute decompensated heart failure

As a therapeutic strategy for patients with ADHF, nesiritide has been evaluated in six randomized controlled clinical trials involving more than 1500 subjects (Table 1). Mills and coworkers [39] performed a multicenter, double-blind,

Table 1
Randomized controlled trials of nesiritide in ADHF

Study	Control	Patients Nesiritide	Control	Nesiritide dose (µg/kg/min)	Median (IQR) duration of infusion (hours)
Mills et al	Placebo	74	29	0.015, 0.03, or 0.06	24.0 (24.0–24.1)
Efficacy trial	Placebo	85	42	0.015 or 0.03	24.2 (7.8–47.7)
Comparative trial	Standard care	203	102	0.015 or 0.03	30.4 (23.0–65.1)
PRECEDENT	Dobutamine	163	83	0.015 or 0.03	24.1 (24.0–46.5)
VMAC	Nitroglycerin or standard care	273	216	0.01	24.3 (24.0–44.2)
PROACTION	Standard care	120	117	0.01	16.9 (12.2–21.9)

Abbreviations: ADHF, acute decompensated heart failure; IQR, interquartile range; PRECEDENT, Prospective Randomized Evaluation of Cardiac Ectopy with Dobutamine or Natrecor Therapy trial; PROACTION, Prospective Randomized Outcomes Study of Acutely Decompensated Congestive Heart Failure Treated Initially as Outpatients with Nesiritide trial; VMAC, Vasodilation in the Management of Acute Congestive Heart Failure trial.
Data from Refs. [25,39,40,41,43].

placebo-controlled evaluation of nesiritide therapy in 103 subjects who had symptomatic heart failure (New York Heart Association [NYHA] class II, III, or IV) and left ventricular systolic dysfunction (left ventricular ejection fraction [LVEF] < 0.35). Subjects were randomized to one of three regimens of nesiritide therapy: 24-hour infusion therapy with nesiritide, 0.015 µg/kg/min, 0.03 µg/kg/min, or 0.06 µg/kg/min versus placebo, with the study drug infusion initiated at least 2 hours after insertion of a pulmonary artery catheter. The primary endpoint was the change from pre- to postinfusion of the study drug on cardiac hemodynamics. When compared with placebo, nesiritide produced significant reductions in PCWP, mean right atrial pressure, and systemic vascular resistance, and significant increases in stroke volume index and cardiac output with no effect on heart rate. These beneficial effects were evident at 1 hour and were sustained throughout the 24-hour infusions. Worsening heart failure necessitating termination of the study drug occurred in 1% of nesiritide versus 17% of control subjects ($P = .014$).

The Efficacy trial was a multicenter, double-blind, placebo-controlled evaluation of nesiritide therapy in 127 subjects with ADHF (94% NYHA class III or IV). This study was likewise guided by measurement of cardiac hemodynamics, and all of the subjects were required to have a systolic blood pressure ≥90 mm Hg, a PCWP ≥18 mm Hg, and a cardiac index ≤ 2.7 L/min/m². Treatment arms consisted of nesiritide, 0.015 µg/kg/min or 0.03 µg/kg/min, or placebo for at least 6 hours. All other parenteral vasoactive agents were withheld during this initial 6-hour period. The primary outcome parameter was the change in PCWP from baseline to 6 hours. Secondary outcomes were global clinical status, clinical symptoms, and other hemodynamic parameters. In this trial, nesiritide produced a dose-dependent decrement in PCWP, right atrial pressure, systemic vascular resistance, and systolic blood pressure, and a moderate increase in cardiac index, but no substantial change in heart rate. Global clinical status as judged by the patient was statistically better for the patients on nesiritide in both the 0.015 µg/kg/min and 0.03 µg/kg/min groups versus the placebo groups ($P < .001$ for the nesiritide versus placebo comparisons). Physician assessments of global status paralleled those of the patients. Dyspnea was improved and fatigue reduced in the nesiritide subjects when compared with the placebo subjects ($P < .001$ for both comparisons) [25].

The Comparative trial was a multicenter, open-label evaluation of nesiritide versus usual therapy in 305 subjects with ADHF (92% NYHA class III or IV). Subjects were randomized to nesiritide, 0.015 µg/kg/min or 0.03 µg/kg/min, or other therapy consisting of a single parenteral vasoactive agent, either an inotrope or other vasodilator, used for the short-term management of ADHF. In all subjects, intravenous diuretics and oral medications could be added at any time. The prespecified primary outcomes were global clinical status and clinical symptoms. In the standard therapy group, 57% of subjects received dobutamine, 19% received milrinone, 18% received nitroglycerin, 6% received dopamine, and 1% received amrinone. Global clinical status, dyspnea, and fatigue improved in all three treatment groups, with no significant differences between treatment groups at 6 hours, 24 hours, and the end of therapy. Weight loss was similar in the three treatment groups; however, intravenous diuretics were required in fewer nesiritide subjects when compared with standard therapy subjects ($P < .001$) [25].

The Prospective Randomized Evaluation of Cardiac Ectopy with Dobutamine or Natrecor Therapy (PRECEDENT) study was a multicenter, open-label, active-controlled evaluation of nesiritide therapy in 255 subjects with ADHF (100% NYHA class III or IV) in which single-agent, intravenous therapy with nesiritide or dobutamine, with or without diuretics, was administered. Subjects were stratified based on the presence or absence of a known history of ventricular tachycardia and were randomized to nesiritide, 0.015 µg/kg/min or 0.03 µg/kg/min, or dobutamine, ≥ 5 µg/kg/min. The minimum infusion duration was 24 hours. All of the patients had three-channel, 24-hour Holter monitor recordings for the 24 hours immediately before (baseline) and after initiation of the study drug. The primary outcome parameters were the changes from baseline in mean heart rate, mean hourly premature ventricular beats, and mean hourly repetitive beats. Secondary outcomes included the frequency of complex ventricular rhythm disturbances. Proarrhythmia was assessed using two established criteria, the Velebit and Cardiac Arrhythmia Pilot Study (CAPS) [40]. At baseline, all three treatment groups had similar heart rates and rates of ventricular ectopy. During treatment, heart rate and ventricular ectopy were increased significantly from baseline in the dobutamine but not the nesiritide subjects. Velebit proarrhythmia criteria were met by 23% of dobutamine versus 2% of nesiritide subjects ($P < 0.001$), and CAPS proarrhythmia criteria were met by 10% of dobutamine versus 0% of nesiritide subjects ($P = .001$) [40].

The Vasodilation in the Management of Acute Congestive Heart Failure (VMAC) trial was a multicenter, double-blind, placebo- and active-controlled evaluation of nesiritide therapy in 489 subjects with ADHF and dyspnea at rest or with minimal activity. Subjects were stratified based on the investigator's decision to measure cardiac hemodynamics with a right-sided heart catheter as part of the management regimen. Patients were then randomized to nesiritide, 0.01 µg/kg/min, in a fixed dose in the noninstrumented patient; a fixed or adjustable-dose nesiritide in the instrumented group; nitroglycerin (adjustable dose); or placebo for the initial 3 hours. After this period, placebo subjects were randomly crossed over to nesiritide (fixed dose) or nitroglycerin therapy. The minimum infusion duration was 24 hours. Primary outcome parameters were the absolute change in PCWP (when applicable) and relief of dyspnea at 3 hours. Secondary outcome parameters included the change in PCWP, relief of dyspnea, and global clinical status at 24 hours. At 3 hours, the mean change in PCWP was -2 mm Hg on placebo therapy, -3.8 mm Hg on nitroglycerin therapy ($P = 0.09$ versus placebo), and -5.8 mm Hg on nesiritide therapy ($P < .001$ versus placebo; $P = 0.03$ versus nitroglycerin). In addition, at 3 hours, nesiritide produced a decrease in dyspnea when compared with placebo ($P = .03$) but not nitroglycerin ($P = .56$). At 24 hours, patients on nesiritide had a significantly greater reduction in PCWP (-8.2 mm Hg) than those on nitroglycerin (-6.3 mm Hg; $P = .04$), with no significant difference in dyspnea ($P = .13$) (Fig. 1) [41].

The Prospective Randomized Outcomes Study of Acutely Decompensated Congestive Heart Failure Treated Initially as Outpatients with Nesiritide (PROACTION) trial was a multicenter, double-blind, placebo-controlled study of nesiritide therapy in 237 emergency department/observation unit patients with ADHF and dyspnea at rest or with minimal activity (walking <20 feet). Patients were randomized to usual care plus nesiritide, 0.01 µg/kg/min, versus usual care plus placebo, with study medication initiated within 3 hours of presentation in the emergency department and continued for a minimum of 12 hours. Standard care was at the investigator's discretion and could include diuretics, oxygen, and one medication or more to reduce systemic vascular resistance and improve cardiac contractility. The primary outcome parameters were the safety profile and clinical effects of nesiritide when added to standard care in the emergency department/observation unit setting. When compared with placebo subjects, subjects who received nesiritide had small statistically insignificant reductions in the requirement for inpatient admission (49% versus 55%; $P = .44$) and mean total hospital length of stay if admitted (5.1 days versus 5.5 days; $P = .62$). Of the subjects admitted, those who received nesiritide had fewer readmissions (10% versus 23%; $P = .06$) and a significantly shorter mean total duration of hospitalization through study day 30 [42]. Eight patients enrolled in the PROACTION trial died from all causes, mostly noncardiac, within 30 days after

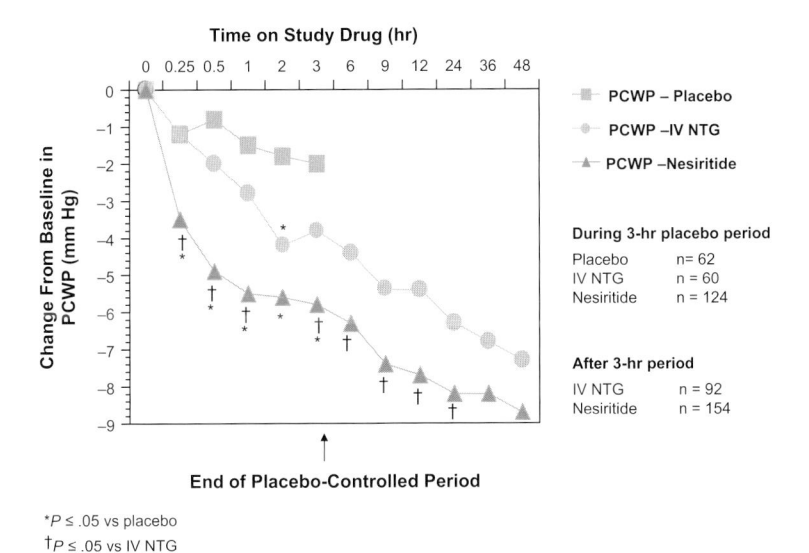

Fig. 1. Hemodynamic effects of nesiritide versus placebo versus intravenous nitroglycerin (IV NTG). (*Data from* Publication Committee for the VMAC Investigators. Intravenous nesiritide vs. nitroglycerin for treatment of decompensated congestive heart failure: a randomized controlled trial. JAMA 2002;287:1531.)

treatment, seven (5.9%) in the nesiritide group and one (0.9%) in the placebo group (HR, 7.03; 95% CI, 0.87–57.15; $P = .066$). A narrowing of the difference in all-cause mortality between the nesiritide and placebo treatment groups was observed at the 180-day time point; 24 patients (20.6%) receiving nesiritide and 20 (17.5%) receiving placebo died (HR, 1.24; 95% CI, 0.68–2.24; $P = .479$) [42,43].

The risk-benefit profile of nesiritide

Resolving questions related to the safety of nesiritide remains an evolutionary process. Similar to other vasodilators, nesiritide produces dose-related hypotension. Because early evaluations of nesiritide used higher than the currently approved starting dose (0.01 μg/kg/min), the frequency and potential complications of this hypotension are difficult to assess, but it is apparent that, with higher doses, the incidence of hypotension increases. In the study by Mills and coworkers, symptomatic hypotension developed in 15% of the patients receiving 0.06 μg/kg/min of nesiritide compared with 5% of those receiving 0.015 μg/kg/min [39]. In the Efficacy trial, 2% and 5% of subjects randomized to nesiritide, 0.015 μg/kg/min and 0.03 μg/kg/min, respectively, experienced symptomatic hypotension versus no patients randomized to placebo ($P = .55$) [25]. In the Comparative trial, the incidence of symptomatic hypotension was higher, occurring in 11% and 17% of patients randomized to nesiritide, 0.015 μg/kg/min and 0.03 μg/kg/min, respectively [25]. In the PRECEDENT study, symptomatic hypotension developed in 17% and 24% of subjects randomized to nesiritide, 0.015 μg/kg/min and 0.03 μg/kg/min, respectively, compared with 2% of subjects randomized to dobutamine ($P < .001$) [40].

In the VMAC trial in which nesiritide was given at a dose of 0.01μg/kg/min, symptomatic hypotension developed in 4% of subjects randomized to nesiritide. In comparison, the incidence of symptomatic hypotension was 5% in patients randomized to nitroglycerin ($P > .99$) [41]. The hypotension noted in the VMAC trial with nesiritide was more troublesome than the hypotension noted with nitroglycerin owing to the longer half-life of nesiritide, 18 versus 3 minutes. Similarly, in the PROACTION trial in which nesiritide was given at a dose of 0.01 μg/kg/min, the frequency of symptomatic hypotension was not significantly different in the nesiritide (2%) and standard care (1%) subjects ($P > .99$) [43]. The degree of blood pressure reduction in subjects receiving nesiritide was related directly to the baseline blood pressure. The greatest reduction in blood pressure occurred in subjects with the greatest degree of baseline hypertension.

Overall, the mean reduction in systolic blood pressure with nesiritide was 1.2 mm Hg, 12.3 mm Hg, and 28.7 mm Hg in subjects with baseline systolic blood pressures less than 101 mm Hg, 101 to 140 mm Hg, and greater than 140 mm Hg, respectively [42].

Nesiritide is associated with an increased risk of acute serum creatinine elevation [44]. This acute increase may be a hemodynamic consequence of blood pressure reduction in patients who are volume depleted or have underlying kidney dysfunction with loss of renal blood flow autoregulatory capability [45,46]. An analysis of five nesiritide trials demonstrated that the risk of an acute increase in serum creatinine was directly related to the prevalence of symptomatic hypotension [47]. An additional observation from the VMAC trial was that nesiritide was not associated with an increased risk of acute serum creatinine elevation in subjects who were receiving low-to-moderate-dose diuretics but was associated with an increase in subjects who were receiving high-dose diuretics, defined as a maximum daily dose of furosemide >160 mg, bumetanide >4 mg, torsemide >80 mg, metolazone >10 mg, chlorothiazide >1000 mg, hydrochlorothiazide >50 mg, or concurrent treatment with two or more of these diuretics regardless of dose [48].

The risk of acute serum creatinine elevation in patients receiving nesiritide is also dose related; consequently, this effect was seen more often in early trials than in later studies [47]. In the VMAC trial, the frequency, onset, and persistence of acute serum creatinine elevations in patients on nesiritide were similar to that in patients on nitroglycerin, and nearly all episodes (approximately 90%) resolved within 30 days of instituting nesiritide or nitroglycerin therapy [41].

The effect of nesiritide on mortality risk is the most troublesome issue and may be difficult to determine definitively given the short duration of nesiritide therapy, numerous potential confounding factors, and low background mortality rates. A pooled analysis of data from three nesiritide trials involving 862 subjects reported that nesiritide may be associated with an increased 30-day mortality risk when compared with other non–inotrope-based control therapies. In this analysis, the 30-day mortality HR for nesiritide therapy after adjusting for study was 1.80 (95% CI, 0.98–3.31; $P = .06$; unadjusted $P = .04$) (Fig. 2) [49]; however, this pooled analysis has several significant limitations that may have influenced the

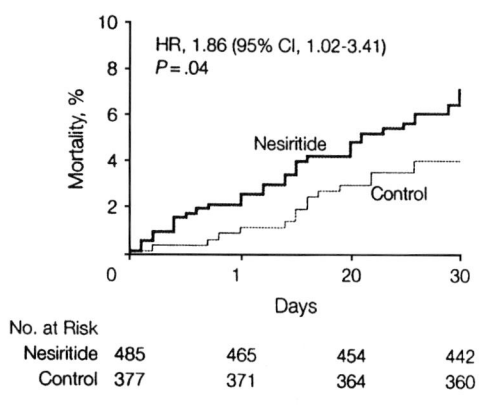

Fig. 2. Kaplan-Meier curves of 30-day mortality associated with control and nesiritide therapies based on nestride study group efficacy trial (NSGET), vasolidation in the management of acute congestive heart failure (VMAC) study, and prospective randomized outcomes study of acutely decompensated congestive heart failure treated initially in outpatients with Natrecor (PROACTION). CI, confidence interval; HR, hazard ratio. (*From* Sackner-Bernstein JD, Kowalski M, Fox M, et al. Short-term risk of death after treatment with nesiritide for decompensated heart failure: a pooled analysis of randomized controlled trials. JAMA 2005; 293(15):1900–5; with permission.)

results. The trials included in this analysis were never designed or powered to assess mortality; consequently, there are substantial differences between studies and between treatment groups within these studies in mortality risk factors, including heart failure severity, the prevalence of acute coronary syndromes, and concomitant therapies. These variables are either uncontrolled or inadequately controlled for in this analysis. In the VMAC trial, which accounts for more than 50% of the subjects in this pooled analysis, there was a significantly greater concomitant use of dobutamine in the subjects randomized to nesiritide compared with nitroglycerin [50], and overall in the three trials used in this 862 patient meta-analysis, inotrope use was greater in subjects randomized to nesiritide when compared with controls before and during study drug infusion [51].

In yet another meta-analysis, the effect on 30-day mortality from acute exposure to nesiritide therapy yielded an HR of 1.34 (95% CI, 0.84–2.15; $P = .22$) and a 6-month HR of 1.05 (95% CI, 0.81–1.36; $P = .73$). These data were pooled from all of the 1507 subjects who participated in randomized controlled clinical trials evaluating nesiritide infusion therapy in patients with ADHF (Table 2) [52]. Neither of these pooled analyses is sufficiently robust to resolve the question, and neither was fully adjusted for baseline differences that may have influenced mortality. It is acknowledged that both analyses appropriately raised the question of risk, but in the absence of prospectively acquired data in a well-designed mortality trial, the question remains unresolved.

An analysis of data from the ADHERE registry involving more than 15,000 patient episodes of ADHF requiring intravenous vasoactive therapy with nesiritide (n = 5220), nitroglycerin (n = 6549), dobutamine (n = 4226), or milrinone (n = 2021) demonstrated that vasodilatory therapy with nesiritide or nitroglycerin was associated with significant reductions in risk-adjusted in-hospital mortality when compared with inotropic therapy with dobutamine or milrinone. There was no significant difference in risk-adjusted mortality between nesiritide and nitroglycerin therapy (Table 3) [18]. Similarly, nesiritide significantly reduced in-hospital mortality risk when compared with milrinone (adjusted OR, 0.24; $P < .001$) or dobutamine (adjusted OR, 0.29; $P < .001$) in a retrospective cohort analysis of data from 2130 patients with ADHF treated with nesiritide (n = 386), milrinone (n = 433), or dobutamine (n = 1311) at 32 academic health centers [53].

Summary and recommendations for therapy

The problem of ADHF represents the next challenge in the evolution of care for patients with left ventricular dysfunction. Clearly, more insight into the pathophysiologic mechanisms that are operative in the conversion from chronic stable heart failure to acute decompensated disease or that provoke acute symptoms in new onset disease is required. The current therapeutic options remain focused on relief of the hemodynamic burden of decompensated heart failure and must be applied in the context of limited data suggesting that the natural history of ADHF can be favorably influenced by medical therapy.

The ideal approach is to address the specific hemodynamic perturbation that is present. The use of diuretics is appropriate for patients with volume overload, the use of vasodilators is appropriate for patients with volume overload and relative hypoperfusion who are not frankly hypotensive, and the use of inotropes is appropriate only for those patients with impending or frank cardiogenic shock. Although it is beyond the scope of this article, aggressive use of evidence-based therapies for chronic heart failure and referral to effective disease management programs should be strongly considered as appropriate treatment strategies for ADHF.

Table 2
Kaplan-Meier estimates of mortality in randomized controlled heart failure trials of nesiritide

Study	Control	30-Day mortality (%) Nesiritide	30-Day mortality (%) Control	180-Day mortality (%) Nesiritide	180-Day mortality (%) Control
Mills et al	Placebo	2.7	7.5	NA	NA
Efficacy trial	Placebo	5.9	4.8	23.1	19.3
Comparative trial	Standard care	6.9	4.9	20.8	23.5
PRECEDENT	Dobutamine	3.7	6.1	16.3	22.2
VMAC	Nitroglycerin standard care	8.1	5.1	25.1	20.8
PROACTION	Standard care	4.2	0.9	NA	NA
FUSION	Standard care	1.4	2.9	9.4	13.5
Pooled (6 studies)[a]		5.9	4.4	NA	NA
Pooled (7 studies)		5.3	4.3	NA	NA
Pooled (4 studies)[a]		NA	NA	21.7	21.5

Abbreviations: FUSION, Follow-Up Serial Infusion of Nesiritide; NA, not applicable; HF, heart failure; PRECEDENT, Prospective Randomized Evaluation of Cardiac Ectopy with Dobutamine or Natrecor Therapy trial; PROACTION, Prospective Randomized Outcomes Study of Acutely Decompensated Congestive Heart Failure Treated Initially as Outpatients with Nesiritide trial; VMAC, Vasodilation in the Management of Acute Congestive Heart Failure trial.

[a] Excludes FUSION.

Adapted from Abraham WT. Nesiritide does not increase 30-day or 6-month mortality risk. Circulation 2005;112(17, Suppl II):676.

Table 3
In-hospital mortality odds ratios for vasoactive therapies in ADHERE

Comparison	Odds ratio[a]	95% Confidence interval
Nesiritide versus		
Nitroglycerin	0.94	0.77–1.16
Dobutamine	0.47	0.39–0.56
Milrinone	0.59	0.48–0.73
Nitroglycerin versus		
Dobutamine	0.46	0.37–0.57
Milrinone	0.69	0.53–0.89
Dobutamine versus		
Milrinone	1.24	1.03–1.55

Abbreviation: ADHERE, Acute Decompensated Heart Failure National Registry.

[a] Adjusted for covariates and propensity score.

Adapted from Abraham WT, Adams KF, Fonarow GC, et al, for the ADHERE Scientific Advisory Committee and Investigators and the ADHERE Study Group. In-hospital mortality in patients with acute decompensated heart failure treated with intravenous vasoactive medications: an analysis from the Acute Decompensated Heart Failure National Registry (ADHERE). J Am Coll Cardiol 2005;46(1):57–64.

When the choice of treatment is vasodilator therapy, nesiritide is a reasonable option. Nesiritide is a synthetic natriuretic peptide with a protean physiologic profile that includes natriuresis, balanced vasodilation, a decrement in filling pressures, an indirect increase in cardiac output, and modulation of neurohormonal activation. Nesiritide remains a US Food and Drug Administration approved treatment option for ADHF. The available data demonstrate a significant effect on elevated filling pressures and at least a moderate effect on the symptom of dyspnea. One should avoid the use of nesiritide in patients with blood pressure lower than 90 mm Hg and administer the drug only at the 0.01 µg/kg/min dose. Additional concern might be expressed if the patient is concomitantly receiving high doses of diuretic therapy. The mortality issues are not resolved. There is neither a clear signal of harm nor benefit. If symptom relief is believed to require vasodilator therapy, the use of nesiritide is an appropriate option. It is hoped that a soon to be commenced 7000 patient mortality trial will resolve the issue of mortality risk. Box 1 includes the new Heart Failure Society of America guidelines for the management of ADHF. Box 2 restates the opinions of the nesiritide review panel regarding the best profile for the use of nesiritide in clinical practice [54].

Box 2. Recommendations of the nesiritide review panel, June 2005

Nesiritide is approved for inpatient management of acute heart failure.
- Use of nesiritide should be limited to patients presenting to the hospital with acute heart failure who have dyspnea at rest.
- Physicians considering the use of nesiritide should consider the following:
Its efficacy in reducing dyspnea
Possible risks of the drug
Availability of alternate therapies to relieve heart failure symptoms

Nesiritide is not recommended for the following:
- Intermittent outpatient infusion
- Scheduled repetitive use
- To improve renal function
- To enhance diuresis

Adapted from Scios, Inc. Panel of cardiology experts provides recommendations to Scios regarding NATRECOR®. Available at: http://sciosinc.com/scios/pr_1118721302. Accessed July 13, 2005.

References

[1] Kozak LJ, Owings MF, Hall MJ. National Hospital Discharge Survey: 2002 annual summary with detailed diagnosis and procedure data. Vital Health Stat 13 2005;158:1–199.

[2] Nieminen MS, Böhm M, Cowie MR, et al. Executive summary of the guidelines on the diagnosis and treatment of acute heart failure: the Task Force on Acute Heart Failure of the European Society of Cardiology. Eur Heart J 2005;26(4):384–416.

[3] Jong P, Vowinckel E, Liu PP, et al. Prognosis and determinants of survival in patients newly hospitalized for heart failure: a population-based study. Arch Intern Med 2002;162:1689–94.

[4] Heart Failure Society of America. Executive Summary: HFSA 2006 comprehensive heart failure practice guideline. J Card Fail 2006;12:10–38.

[5] Fonarow GC, for the ADHERE Scientific Advisory Committee. The Acute Decompensated Heart

Failure National Registry (ADHERE): opportunities to improve care of patients hospitalized with acute decompensated heart failure. Rev Cardiovasc Med 2003;4(Suppl 7):S21–30.
[6] The ESCAPE Investigators and ESCAPE Study Coordinators. Evaluation study of congestive heart failure and pulmonary artery catheterization effectiveness: the ESCAPE trial. JAMA 2005;294: 1625–33.
[7] Emerman CL, DeMarco T, Costanzo MR, et al, for the ADHERE Scientific Advisory Committee. Impact of intravenous diuretics on the outcomes of patients hospitalized with acute decompensated heart failure: insights from the ADHERE Registry [abstract 368]. J Card Fail 2004;10(Suppl 4):S116.
[8] Ikram H, Chan W, Espiner EA, et al. Haemodynamic and hormone responses to acute and chronic furosemide therapy in congestive heart failure. Clin Sci 1980;59(6):443–9.
[9] Gottlieb SS, Brater DC, Thomas I, et al. BG9719 (CVT-124), an A_1 adenosine receptor antagonist, protects against the decline in renal function observed with diuretic therapy. Circulation 2002; 105(11):1348–53.
[10] Francis GS, Siegel RM, Goldsmith SR, et al. Acute vasoconstrictor response to intravenous furosemide in patients with chronic congestive heart failure: activation of the neurohumoral axis. Ann Intern Med 1985;103(1):1–6.
[11] Domanski M, Norman J, Pitt B, et al. Diuretic use, progressive heart failure, and death in patients in the studies of left ventricular dysfunction (SOLVD). J Am Coll Cardiol 2003;42(4):705–8.
[12] Cooper HA, Dries DL, Davis CE, et al. Diuretics and risk of arrhythmic death in patients with left ventricular dysfunction. Circulation 1999;100(12): 1311–5.
[13] Ellison DH. Diuretic drugs and the treatment of edema from clinic to bench and back again. Am J Kidney Dis 1994;23(5):623–43.
[14] Costanzo MR. UNLOAD: Ultrafiltration vs. IV Diuretics for Patients Hospitalized for Acute Decompensated Congestive Heart Failure. Late Breaking Clinical Trials. Presented at the ACC Scientific Meeting. Atlanta, March 14, 2006.
[15] Cuffe MS, Califf RM, Adams KF, et al. OPTIME-CHF [outcomes of a prospective trial of intravenous milrinone for exacerbations of chronic heart failure]. Short-term intravenous milrinone for acute exacerbation of chronic heart failure. A randomized controlled trial. JAMA 2002;287:1541–7.
[16] Stiles S. SURVIVE: no levosimendan survival benefit over dobutamine in acute HF. Available at: http://www.theheart.org. Accessed August 7, 2006.
[17] Stiles S. REVIVE-2: levosimendan improves five-day clinical status in acute HF. Available at: http://www.theheart.org. Accessed August 7, 2006.
[18] Abraham WT, Adams KF, Fonarow GC, et al. The ADHERE Scientific Advisory Committee and Investigators and the ADHERE Study Group. In-hospital mortality in patients with acute decompensated heart failure treated with intravenous vasoactive medications: an analysis from the Acute Decompensated Heart Failure National Registry (ADHERE). J Am Coll Cardiol 2005; 46(1):57–64.
[19] Ferreira A, Bettencourt P, Dias P, et al. Neurohormonal activation, the renal dopaminergic system and sodium handling in patients with severe heart failure under vasodilator therapy. Clin Sci 2001; 100(5):557–66.
[20] Keating GM, Goa KL. Nesiritide: a review of its use in acute decompensated heart failure. Drugs 2003; 63(1):47–70.
[21] Boerrigter G, Burnett JC Jr. Recent advances in natriuretic peptides in congestive heart failure. Expert Opin Investig Drugs 2004;13(6):643–52.
[22] Abraham WT, Lowes BD, Ferguson DA, et al. Systemic hemodynamic, neurohormonal, and renal effects of a steady-state infusion of human brain natriuretic peptide in patients with hemodynamically decompensated heart failure. J Card Fail 1998;4(1):37–44.
[23] Marcus LS, Hart D, Packer M, et al. Hemodynamic and renal excretory effects of human brain natriuretic peptide infusion in patients with congestive heart failure: a double-blind, placebo-controlled, randomized crossover trial. Circulation 1996; 94(12):3184–9.
[24] Michaels AD, Klein A, Madden JA, et al. Effects of intravenous nesiritide on human coronary vasomotor regulation and myocardial oxygen uptake. Circulation 2003;107(21):2697–701.
[25] Colucci WS, Elkayam U, Horton DP, et al, for the Nesiritide Study Group. Intravenous nesiritide, a natriuretic peptide, in the treatment of decompensated congestive heart failure. N Engl J Med 2000;343(4): 246–53.
[26] Brunner-La Rocca HP, Kaye DM, Woods RL, et al. Effects of intravenous brain natriuretic peptide on regional sympathetic activity in patients with chronic heart failure as compared with healthy control subjects. J Am Coll Cardiol 2001;37(5):1221–7.
[27] Cataliotti A, Boerrigter G, Costello-Boerrigter LC, et al. Brain natriuretic peptide enhances renal actions of furosemide and suppresses furosemide-induced aldosterone activation in experimental heart failure. Circulation 2004;109(13):1680–5.
[28] Aronson D, Burger AJ. Effect of nesiritide (human b-type natriuretic peptide) and dobutamine on heart rate variability in decompensated heart failure. Am Heart J 2004;148(5):920–6.
[29] Pitt B, Zannad F, Remme WJ, et al. The effect of spironolactone on morbidity and mortality in patients with severe heart failure. N Engl J Med 1999;341: 709–17.
[30] Pitt B, Remme WJ, Zannad F, et al. Eplerenone, a selective aldosterone blocker, in patients with left

ventricular dysfunction after myocardial infarction. N Engl J Med 2003;348:1309–21.
[31] Yancy CW. Treatment with B-type natriuretic peptide for chronic decompensated heart failure: insights learned from the follow-up serial infusion of nesiritide (FUSION) trial. Heart Failure Reviews 2004;9(3[special issue]):209–16.
[32] Aronson D, Burger AJ. Intravenous nesiritide (human B-type natriuretic peptide) reduces plasma endothelin-1 levels in patients with decompensated congestive heart failure. Am J Cardiol 2002;90(4): 435–8.
[33] Holmes SJ, Espiner EA, Richards AM, et al. Renal, endocrine, and hemodynamic effects of human brain natriuretic peptide in normal man. J Clin Endocrinol Metab 1993;76(1):91–6.
[34] Jensen KT, Carstens J, Pedersen EB. Effect of BNP on renal hemodynamics, tubular function and vasoactive hormones in humans. Am J Physiol 1998; 274(1 Pt 2):F63–72.
[35] Jensen KT, Eiskjaer H, Carstens J, et al. Renal effects of brain natriuretic peptide in patients with congestive heart failure. Clin Sci (Lond) 1999;96(1):5–15.
[36] Akabane S, Matsushima Y, Matsuo H, et al. Effects of brain natriuretic peptide on renin secretion in normal and hypertonic saline-infused kidney. Eur J Pharmacol 1991;198(2–3):143–8.
[37] Wang DJ, Dowling TC, Meadows D, et al. Nesiritide does not improve renal function in patients with chronic heart failure and worsening serum creatinine. Circulation 2004;110(12):1620–5.
[38] Elkayam U, Singh H, Akhter MW, et al. Effects of intravenous nesiritide on renal hemodynamics in patients with congestive heart failure [abstract 256]. J Card Fail 2004;10(Suppl 4):S88.
[39] Mills RM, LeJemtel TH, Horton DP, et al. On behalf of the Natrecor Study Group. Sustained hemodynamic effects of an infusion of nesiritide (human B-type natriuretic peptide) in heart failure: a randomized, double-blind, placebo-controlled clinical trial. J Am Coll Cardiol 1999;34(1):155–62.
[40] Burger AJ, Horton DP, LeJemtel T, et al. Effect of nesiritide (B-type natriuretic peptide) and dobutamine on ventricular arrhythmias in the treatment of patients with acutely decompensated congestive heart failure: the PRECEDENT Study. Am Heart J 2002;144(6):1102–8.
[41] Publication Committee for the VMAC Investigators. Intravenous nesiritide vs. nitroglycerin for treatment of decompensated congestive heart failure: a randomized controlled trial. JAMA 2002; 287(12):1531–40.
[42] Peacock WF IV, Emerman CL, Silver MA, et al. Nesiritide added to standard care favorably reduces systolic blood pressure compared with standard care alone in patients with acute decompensated heart failure. Am J Emerg Med 2005;23(3):327–31.
[43] Peacock WF, Holland R, Gyarmathy R, et al. Observation unit treatment of heart failure with nesiritide: results from the PROACTION trial. J Emerg Med 2005;29(3):243–52.
[44] Sackner-Bernstein JD, Skopicki HA, Aaronson KD. Risk of worsening renal function with nesiritide in patients with acutely decompensated heart failure. Circulation 2005;111(12):1487–91.
[45] Epstein BJ. Elevations in serum creatinine concentration: concerning or reassuring? Pharmacotherapy 2004;24(5):697–702.
[46] Butler J, Forman DE, Abraham WT, et al. Relationship between heart failure treatment and development of worsening renal function among hospitalized patients. Am Heart J 2004;147(2): 331–8.
[47] Abraham WT. Serum creatinine elevations in patients receiving nesiritide are related to starting dose [abstract 2789]. Circulation 2005;112(17, Suppl II):589.
[48] Heywood JT. Combining nesiritide with high-dose diuretics may increase the risk of increased serum creatinine [abstract 240]. J Card Fail 2005;11(Suppl 6):S154.
[49] Sackner-Bernstein JD, Kowalski M, Fox M, et al. Short-term risk of death after treatment with nesiritide for decompensated heart failure: a pooled analysis of randomized controlled trials. JAMA 2005; 293(15):1900–5.
[50] Gortney JS, Porter KB. Risk of death with nesiritide. JAMA 2005;294(8):897–8.
[51] Burger AJ. Risk of death with nesiritide. JAMA 2005;294(8):897.
[52] Abraham WT. Nesiritide does not increase 30-day or 6-month mortality risk. Circulation 2005; 112(17, Suppl II):676.
[53] Arnold LM, Carroll NV, Oinonen M, et al. Mortality and length of hospital stay in patients receiving dobutamine, milrinone, or nesiritide for acute decompensated heart failure. J Card Fail 2004; 10(Suppl 4):S103.
[54] Scios, Inc. Available at: http://www.sciosinc.com/scios/pr_1118721302. Accessed July 13, 2005.

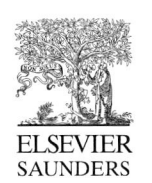

Therapeutic Potential for Existing and Novel Forms of Natriuretic Peptides

Horng H. Chen, MBBCh*, John C. Burnett Jr, MD

Mayo Clinic College of Medicine, Rochester, MN, USA

The natriuretic peptides are a family of peptides, each with a 17–amino acid disulfide ring structure, that are genetically distinct with diverse actions in cardiovascular, renal, and endocrine homeostasis [1]. In humans, the family consists of atrial natriuretic peptide (ANP) and brain natriuretic peptide (BNP) of myocardial cell origin, C-type natriuretic peptide (CNP) of endothelial origin, and urodilatin (Uro) thought to be derived from the kidney [2,3]. The 126–amino acid ANP prohormone also gives rise to three other fragment peptides: long-acting natriuretic peptide (LANP) (amino acids 1–30), vessel dilator (amino acids 31–67), and kaliuretic peptide (amino acids 79–98) [4]. There are also recent reports of novel forms of BNP, notably albuBNP [5], which is a human recombinant fusion hormone of BNP and human albumin and oral BNP using proprietary technology consisting of short amphiphilic oligomers covalently attached to BNP [6]. Furthermore, natriuretic peptides have been isolated from a range of other vertebrates. Notably, some have been found in snake venoms. Dendroaspis auguticeps natriuretic peptide (DNP) was detected in the venom of *Dendroaspis auguticeps* (the green mamba) [7]. CNP analogues were cloned from the venom glands of snakes of the Crotalinae subfamily [8]. Pseudocerastes persicus natriuretic peptide (PNP) was isolated from the venom of the Iranian snake *Pseudocerastes persicus* [9], and three natriuretic-like peptides (TNP-a, TNP-b, and TNP-c) were isolated from the venom of *Oxyuranus microlepidotus* [10].

Human recombinant ANP (carperitide) has been approved for the clinical management of acute decompensated congestive heart failure (CHF) in Japan since 1995 [11]. Human recombinant BNP (nesiritide) has been approved by the Food and Drug Administration (FDA) for the same clinical indication in the United States since 2001 [12]. Human recombinant Uro (ularitide) is currently undergoing phase III clinical trails in Europe [2].

This review provides an update on important issues regarding the therapeutic potential of existing and novel forms of natriuretic peptides beyond acute decompensated heart failure.

Physiologic properties of the natriuretic peptides and their therapeutic potential

ANP, BNP, and Uro bind to the natriuretic peptide-A receptor (NPR-A), which, via $3',5'$-cyclic guanosine monophosphate (cGMP), mediates natriuresis, vasodilatation, renin inhibition, and anti-ischemic, anti-mitogenesis, and positive lusitropism [1]. CNP lacks natriuretic actions but possesses vasodilating and growth-inhibiting actions via the guanylyl cyclase–linked natriuretic peptide-B receptor (NPR-B) [13]. All four peptides are cleared by the natriuretic peptide-C receptor (NPR-C) and degraded by the ectoenzyme neutral endopeptidase 24.11 (NEP), both of which are widely expressed in kidney, lung, and vascular wall [14]. These physiologic

---

This research was supported by grants PO1 HL 76611 and HL 36634 from the National Institutes of Health, the Mayo Foundation, and an American Heart Association Scientist Development Grant awarded to Dr. Chen.

* Corresponding author. Cardiorenal Research Laboratory, Guggenheim 915, Mayo Clinic and Foundation, 200 First Street SW, Rochester, MN 55905.

E-mail address: chen.horng@mayo.edu (H.H. Chen).

properties of the natriuretic peptides are discussed elsewhere in detail. Currently, the natriuretic peptides are approved for the management of acute decompensated heart failure; however, their therapeutic potential extends beyond this indication and includes the following:

- Chronic therapy for chronic heart failure and hypertension
- Prevention of post myocardial infarction adverse left ventricular remodeling
- Renal protection during cardiopulmonary bypass surgeries
- Therapy for asthma
- Therapy for cancer

Chronic therapy for chronic heart failure and hypertension

The concept of chronic administration of natriuretic peptides, particularly in delaying the progression of heart failure and hypertension, is beginning to emerge. This concept is based on studies suggesting that inadequate production of BNP may occur in heart failure [15] and hypertension [16], as well as recent evidence suggesting that there may be altered molecular forms of BNP, with reduced biologic activity of BNP in advanced heart failure with an actual absence of the biologically active BNP-32 [17]. The paradigm of chronic peptide therapy in human disease is not new. Diabetes is such a paradigm wherein inadequate production of the protein insulin requires chronic administration of synthetic insulin to maintain optimal metabolic balance.

Chen and coworkers recently addressed the concept of defining the cardiorenal and humoral actions of repeated short-term administration of subcutaneous BNP during the evolution of experimental heart failure [15]. They used a unique large animal model of heart failure that mimicked human asymptomatic left ventricular dysfunction (ALVD). They found that plasma BNP and cGMP rapidly increased after acute subcutaneous BNP administration with increases in urinary sodium excretion, urine flow, and renal blood flow in association with reductions in cardiac filling pressures. After 10 days of repeated short-term administration of subcutaneous BNP, cardiac output was increased, and systemic vascular resistance and pulmonary capillary wedge pressure were decreased in a comparison with untreated dogs with heart failure (Fig. 1). This study demonstrated for the first time that repeated short-term administration of subcutaneous BNP during the evolution of experimental ALVD results in an improvement of cardiovascular hemodynamics, supporting the concept of novel chronic administration of BNP in the therapeutics of heart failure.

This experimental study in an animal model of evolving heart failure was followed by a study to assess the safety and efficacy of repeated doses of subcutaneous BNP in human New York Heart Association (NYHA) class II to III CHF [18]. This short-term, 3-day study defined the cardiorenal and humoral responses to subcutaneous BNP administered every 12 hours with a total of five doses over 72 hours in a single-blind, placebo-controlled design [19]. The initial saline placebo resulted in no change in measured parameters. The first dose of BNP increased cardiac output and reduced systolic blood pressure without a change in heart rate. Plasma BNP and urinary cGMP excretion increased with natriuresis and diuresis. Plasma renin activity and aldosterone decreased. These favorable biologic responses were observed with the fifth dose 3 days after the initial dose. The investigators concluded that subcutaneous administration of BNP in human CHF has efficacy and safety, warranting further investigations with a goal of attempting to delay the progression of heart failure by focusing on earlier stages of heart failure with a kidney that is highly responsive to the cardiac peptide BNP. Chen and coworkers are currently conducting a double-blind, placebo-controlled study to determine the effects of 8 weeks of chronic subcutaneous BNP administration on left ventricular volumes in patients who have CHF.

AlbuBNP is a long-acting form of BNP produced by recombinant fusion to human serum albumin [5]. Completed studies have assessed the bioactivities of AlbuBNP by a NPR-A–mediated cGMP activation assay, hemodynamic responses, and plasma cGMP elevation. The pharmacokinetic properties were determined after single intravenous or subcutaneous bolus injection in C57/BL6 mice. AlbuBNP had approximately the same maximal bioactivity as BNP to activate cGMP in the in vitro NPR-A/cGMP assay. The EC_{50s} were 28.4 ± 1.2 and 0.46 ± 1.1 nM for AlbuBNP and BNP, respectively. AlbuBNP lowered systolic and diastolic blood pressure in spontaneously hypertensive rats, with sustainable mean arterial pressure reduction for more than 2 days. The elimination half-life in mice was dramatically increased from 3 minutes for BNP to 12 to 19

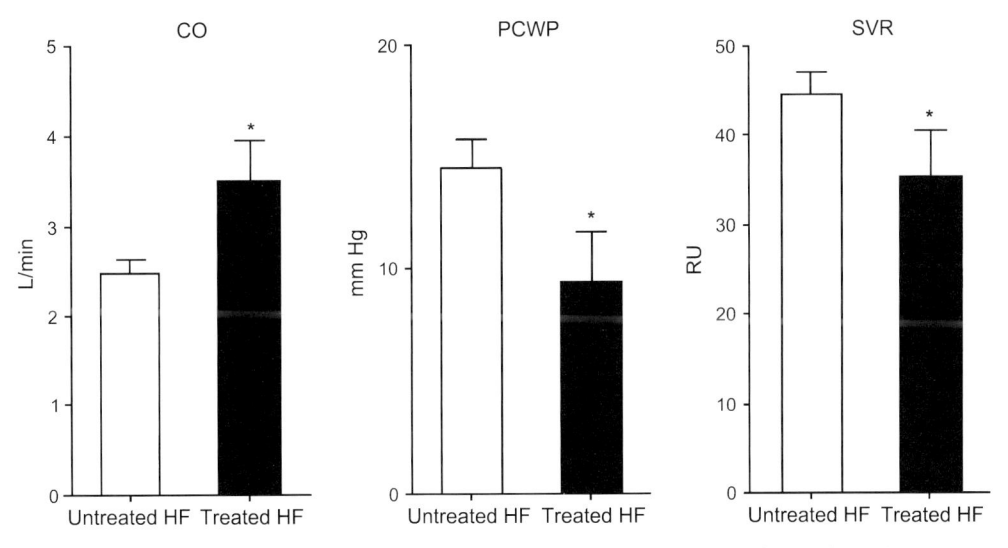

Fig. 1. Cardiac output (CO), pulmonary capillary wedge pressure (PCWP), and systemic vascular resistance (SVR) of the dogs in the chronic subcutaneous BNP group (treated heart failure) on day 11 of rapid ventricular pacing compared with dogs with untreated heart failure on day 11 of rapid ventricular pacing. *$P < .05$ versus untreated heart failure. HF, heart failure. (*From* Chen HH, Grantham JA, Schirger JA, et al. Subcutaneous administration of brain natriuretic peptide in experimental heart failure. J Am Coll Cardiol 2000;36:1706; with permission.)

hours for AlbuBNP; therefore, AlbuBNP is bioactive and has desired pharmacokinetic properties for long-term use. It has the potential to be developed as a new therapeutic option for chronic, acute, and post-acute CHF to alleviate symptoms, improve clinical status, and slow the disease progression by sustained drug exposure via infrequent simple subcutaneous injections.

Cataliotti and coworkers advanced an exciting concept, that is, the development and use of an orally available human BNP (Fig. 2), and reported the feasibility and biologic activity of oral BNP using proprietary technology employing short amphiphilic oligomers covalently attached to BNP [6]. Oral BNP increased plasma BNP, activated plasma cGMP, and reduced mean arterial pressure in conscious normal dogs. Although BNP is an important intravenous drug in treating hospitalized patients with acute decomposition, an oral dosage form may broaden the application of this therapy to patients with various stages in the progression of heart failure and be an important preventive strategy in evolving heart failure. Because of its antifibrotic actions and blood pressure–lowering properties, the use of oral BNP as a therapeutic agent for human heart hypertension and heart failure warrants further research.

Prevention of adverse left ventricular remodeling post myocardial infarction

Acute myocardial infarction is a complication of coronary artery disease and may lead to loss of ventricular myocardium with cardiac enlargement and fibrosis. Post acute myocardial infarction left ventricular remodeling begins within hours of the acute event with permanent consequences [20]. Previous studies have demonstrated that left

Fig. 2. Structure of oral BNP. (*From* Cataliotti A, Schirger JA, Martin FL, et al. Oral human brain natriuretic peptide activates cyclic guanosine 3′,5′-monophosphate and decreases mean arterial pressure. Circulation 2005;112:836; with permission.)

ventricular remodeling is one of the major determinants of long-term survival post acute myocardial infarction [21].

The role of the natriuretic peptides in cardiac remodeling is discussed in detail elsewhere in this issue. Recent studies have reported that the natriuretic peptides have direct antifibrotic and antiproliferative effects on the myocardium. Furthermore, it has been demonstrated that the natriuretic peptides suppress the sympathetic nervous system, renin-angiotensin-aldosterone system (RAAS), and endothelin system, all of which stimulate left ventricular remodeling [22]. More importantly, it has been reported that in the acute phase of myocardial infarction, the secretion of the cardiac natriuretic peptides may be insufficient relative to the chronic phase [23,24]; therefore, augmentation of the cardiac natriuretic peptide system, such as by exogenous administration of peptide, may prevent post acute myocardial infarction left ventricular remodeling because of the cardioprotective effects. This possibility has led to a study by Hayashi and coworkers [25] who reported that intravenous ANP prevented adverse left ventricular remodeling in patients with first anterior acute myocardial infarction. In that study, 60 patients with a first anterior acute myocardial infarction were randomly divided into the ANP (n = 30) or nitroglycerin (GTN) (n = 30) groups after direct percutaneous transluminal coronary angioplasty (PTCA). The left ventricular ejection fraction (LVEF), end-diastolic volume index (LVEDVI), and end-systolic volume index (LVESVI) were evaluated at the acute phase and after 1 month. The LVEF was significantly improved after 1 month when compared with the baseline value in both groups, but it was improved more in the ANP group than in the GTN group (54.6 ± 1.1%, 50.8 ± 1.3%, $P < .05$). Left ventricular enlargement was prevented in the ANP group (LVEDVI, 85.8 ± 3.1 mL/m^2 to 87.3 ± 2.7 mL/m^2, P = NS; LVESVI, 45.6 ± 1.8 mL/m^2 to 41.0 ± 2.1 mL/m^2, $P < .05$) but not in the GTN group (LVEDVI, 86.2 ± 4.1 to 100.2 ± 3.7, $P < .01$; LVESVI, 46.3 ± 2.8 mL/m^2 to 51.1 ± 3.0 mL/m^2, P = NS). During the infusion, ANP suppressed plasma levels of aldosterone, angiotensin II, and endothelin-1 when compared with GTN.

Based on the results of the study, the Japan-Working groups of acute myocardial Infarction for the reduction of Necrotic Damage by ANP (J-WIND-ANP) designed a prospective, randomized, multicenter study to evaluate whether ANP as an adjunctive therapy for acute myocardial infarction reduces myocardial infarct size and improves regional wall motion [26]. Twenty hospitals in Japan will participate in the J-WIND-ANP study. Patients with acute myocardial infarction who are candidates for PTCA will be randomly allocated to receive intravenous ANP or a placebo. The primary endpoints are (1) estimated infarct size (creatine kinase and troponin T) and (2) left ventricular function (left ventriculograms). Single nucleotide polymorphisms that may be associated with the function of ANP and the susceptibility of acute myocardial infarction will be examined.

One of the limitations of the Hayashi study is that angiotensin-coverting enzyme inhibitor (ACEI) was withheld during the 72 hours of ANP infusion, which is in contradiction to American College of Cardiology/American Heart Association guidelines. For ACE inhibition in the management of acute anterior ST-elevation myocardial infarction (STEMI), the guidelines state [27], "An ACE inhibitor should be administered orally within the first 24 hours of STEMI to patients with anterior infarction without known contraindications to that class of medications." Moreover, despite the structural similarity between ANP and BNP, BNP is emerging as the more potent peptide, with greater cardiorenal and humoral actions and less susceptibility to degradation by neutral endopeptidase 24-11 [6,28,29]. Chen and coworkers [30] have completed a pilot study (n = 24) and determined that 72 hours of intravenous BNP at 0.006 µg/kg/min in addition to standard therapy including ACEI is tolerable and has favorable effects on left ventricular remodeling. Based on the results of the pilot study, Chen and colleagues are currently conducting a double-blind, placebo-controlled study to determine the effects of 72 hours of BNP infusion, 0.006 µg/kg/min, on left ventricular remodeling post anterior STEMI.

Renal protection during cardiopulmonary bypass surgery

Mild-to-moderate renal insufficiency is associated with increased morbidity and mortality post cardiopulmonary bypass cardiac surgery [31]. Specifically, there is an increased likelihood of postoperative mechanical renal support, a longer length of hospital stay, and higher in-hospital mortality [32]. The incidence of acute renal failure as defined by the doubling of plasma creatinine after cardiac surgery has been reported to range from 5% to 30%, with the highest incidence in patients with baseline renal insufficiency (creatinine clearance <60 mL/min) preoperatively [33]. The beneficial renal actions of natriuretic peptides include increases in renal blood flow and glomerular filtration rate resulting in natriuresis and diuresis. Unlike conventional diuretics that activate the RAAS, natriuretic peptides inhibit the RAAS despite marked natriuresis and diuresis [28]. Although preclinical and early clinical studies have demonstrated the renal enhancing effects of systemic intravenous administration of BNP, the clinical trials that led to the FDA approval of nesiritide for the management of acute CHF have been conflicting with regards to the renal enhancing properties of nesiritide. Specifically, a recent study reported that intravenous nesiritide did not improve renal function in 15 patients with worsening renal function in response to furosemide [34]. Furthermore, a meta-analysis of the clinical trials suggested that nesiritide might be detrimental to renal function in patients with acute decompensated CHF [35].

The discrepancy in the renal actions of nesiritide reported is most likely multifactorial; however one potential explanation emerges. Critical review of the preclinical [6], early clinical [36–38], and clinical studies suggests that the lack of renal effects of nesiritide in some of the clinical studies may be due in part to the fact that the doses used in the clinical studies resulted in significantly decreased blood pressure and, hence, renal perfusion pressure. Supporting this hypothesis is a study by Chen and coworkers in experimental CHF, which demonstrated that a low dose of subcutaneously administered BNP, which did not lower blood pressure, had a more beneficial renal hemodynamic profile than a higher dose that lowered blood pressure [15]. Furthermore, Riter and coworkers [39] have recently completed a retrospective study suggesting that the use of nonhypotensive low-dose nesiritide with low-dose furosemide therapy in acute decompensated CHF patients with renal dysfunction improved renal function as compared with standard-dose nesiritide, which resulted in the decrease in blood pressure. This hypothesis is further supported by the fact that while earlier studies with high-dose ANP did not demonstrate beneficial renal actions, low-dose intravenous ANP infusion has been shown to improve the glomerular filtration rate and creatinine clearance in patients post cardiopulmonary bypass cardiac surgery [40].

Valsson and coworkers also reported the effects of intravenous infusion of ANP on renal function in patients with acute heart failure and renal impairment after cardiac surgery. Twelve patients (mean age, 68 years; range, 44–78 years) treated with inotropic drugs and an intra-aortic balloon pump (n = 8) were studied 1 to 3 days after cardiac surgery. Patients had acute renal impairment defined as a rise in serum creatinine of more than 50% compared with preoperative values. Patients were receiving dopamine and furosemide infusion to increase urine flow. Baseline measurements of the glomerular filtration rate and renal blood flow (51Cr-EDTA and PAH clearance) were first performed during two 30-minute periods. ANP was then administered for two consecutive 30-minute periods (25 and 50 ng/kg/min), followed by two control periods. Urine flow, the glomerular filtration rate, and renal blood flow increased 62%, 43%, and 38%, respectively, whereas renal vascular resistance decreased 30%. It was concluded that ANP improved renal function and decreased elevated renal vascular resistance in patients with renal dysfunction after cardiac surgery. The improvement in renal blood flow and glomerular filtration rate may be of potential therapeutic value to prevent or treat exaggerated renal vasoconstriction in patients with acute renal impairment following cardiac surgery [33].

Recently, the preliminary results of the Nesiritide Administered Peri-Anesthesia in Patients Undergoing Cardiothoracic Surgery (NAPA) trial were presented in abstract format [41]. The objective of the study was to evaluate the impact of perioperative nesiritide infusion on post coronary artery bypass graft renal function. The study enrolled 303 heart failure patients in the United States, all of whom had a LVEF ≤40% and NYHA class II-IV symptoms. Subjects were randomized to nesiritide, 0.01 µg/kg/min (no bolus), or placebo after the induction of anesthesia and remained on nesiritide for 24 to 96 hours. Postoperative renal dysfunction, defined as an increase in serum creatinine > 0.5 mg/dL by hospital discharge or hospital day 14 (whichever came first), occurred in 30 of 134 patients (22%) in the placebo group versus 12 of 137 patients (9%) in the nesiritide group ($P = .002$). In addition, the peak increase in serum creatinine was lower in nesiritide-treated patients (0.16 ± 0.03 versus 0.33 ± 0.04; $P = .001$), 24-hour urine output was greater (2.9 versus 2.4 L, $P < .001$), and there was a reduction in hospital length of stay (9.1 versus 11.4 days, $P = .043$) with no difference in adverse events, including mortality.

The Mayo Clinic Group has recently completed a double-blind, placebo-controlled pilot study in patients (n = 40) with renal insufficiency preoperatively (defined by having a calculated creatinine clearance [CrCl] of <50 mL/min determined by the Cockroft-Gault formula) undergoing cardiac surgery with cardiopulmonary bypass. Patients were randomized to placebo (n = 20) or intravenous low-dose nesiritide (n = 20), 0.005 μg/kg/min for 24 hours, started after the induction of anesthesia and before cardiopulmonary bypass. These results will be presented at the upcoming American Heart Association annual scientific meeting in 2006. Further studies are warranted to determine whether these physiologic observations can be translated into differences in patient outcomes.

Therapy for asthma

The hallmarks of asthma are bronchoconstriction and airway inflammation in response to allergens, viruses, and pollutants. Natriuretic peptides levels are significantly increased during severe asthma attacks. Furthermore, natriuretic peptides have been localized in peripheral lung tissue, tracheal epithelial cells, respiratory epithelium, human fetal lung tissue, pulmonary veins, and striated muscle cells, suggesting that natriuretic peptides might have an important role in the biologic activities of the lung [42]. Lung cells express the guanylyl cyclase–coupled NPR-A and the guanylyl cyclase–uncoupled receptor NPR-C [43]. The natriuretic peptide system in the lung has several biologic activities, such as vasodilatation, bronchorelaxation, pulmonary permeability, and surfactant production and action [44]. The bronchodilatory activity of natriuretic peptides is based on their stimulation of intracellular cGMP as an alternative pathway to β_2-agonists such as albuterol, the current first-line bronchodilator, which interacts with smooth bronchial muscle by increasing the intracellular concentration of cyclic adenosine monophosphate (cAMP), inducing bronchodilation. Lung tissue–specific expression of natriuretic peptides is controlled by a number of factors, including glucocorticoids, thyroid hormone, hemodynamic overload, and hydration status [45]. Furthermore, the natriuretic peptide system seems to affect lymphoid organs greatly, such as the thymus, and the development of immunity and tolerance to diverse antigens [46].

ANP induces relaxation of pulmonary arteries and dilates the trachea and bronchi in humans and various animal species. Intravenous ANP inhibits antigen-induced bronchoconstriction in ovalbumin-induced asthma in guinea pigs [47]. In humans, exogenous ANP reverses airway hyperreactivity when given intravenously or by inhalation and has also been shown to modify bronchial reactivity to inhaled histamine, propanolol, and nebulized water. Specifically, Angus and coworkers [48] demonstrated that intravenous ANP had a bronchodilator effect comparable with that of inhaled albuterol in a randomized double-blind cross-over study. In contrast, Fluge and coworkers [49] showed that intravenous ANP produced only a 50% bronchodilator effect when compared with salbutamol.

BNP has also been shown to have a potent bronchodilator effect when administered intravenously in guinea pigs [47]. Recently, Ackerman and coworkers [50] reported the findings of a prospective, open-label study of eight patients investigating the bronchodilator effect of recombinant human BNP, nesiritide, on patients with asthma. After 180 minutes of nesiritide infusion, the following measurements showed significant changes: forced expiratory volume in 1 s (FEV_1) increased to 2.41 ± 0.78 L (mean increase, 520 mL; $P = .012$) and forced vital capacity (FVC) increased to 3.65 ± 1.05 L (mean increase, 630 mL; $P = .017$).

Urodilatin has been shown to exhibit airway-relaxing effects in vitro using tracheal muscle strips. In vivo experiments in rodents and in patients with mild asthma confirmed these results [49]. A randomized, double-blind, placebo-controlled clinical phase II study with cross-over design using intravenous infusions of urodilatin at various doses showed beneficial effects in patients sustaining bronchial asthma. Urodilatin increased FEV_1, maximal vital capacity, peak expiratory flow, and maximal expiratory flow at 75% (MEF_{75}), 50% (MEF_{50}), and 25% (MEF_{25}) of FVC at infusion doses of 10, 30, or 60 ng/kg/min. Optimal effects were observed at urodilatin doses of 30 and 60 ng/kg/min. Urodilatin monotherapy shows a bronchodilation comparable with that induced by a standard dose of albuterol. Urodilatin infusion combined with albuterol inhalation results in a significantly stronger bronchodilatory effect compared with that obtained by monotherapy with either drug [51].

Further studies are required to determine whether these physiologic findings with ANP, BNP, and urodilatin will translate to improved clinical outcome in patients with asthma.

Therapy for cancer

Studies are undergoing to define the ability of the natriuretic peptides to inhibit the growth of cancers. Specifically, ANP and the three other fragment peptides, LANP, vessel dilator, and kaliuretic peptide, have been employed in in vitro and in vivo preclinical studies. The mechanism by which the natriuretic peptides decrease cancer cell number and the reason for their antiproliferative effects is the inhibition of DNA synthesis [52]. Cell cycle progression of cancer cells is directly affected by several of the natriuretic peptides. Vesely and coworkers [52] first reported that vessel dilator, LANP, kaliuretic peptide, and ANP at concentrations of 1 mmol/L decreased the number of human pancreatic adenocarcinoma cells in culture by 65%, 47%, 37%, and 34%, respectively, within 24 hours. This decrease was sustained without any proliferation of the adenocarcinoma cells occurring in the 3 days following this decrease in number studied in vitro. Subsequently, these investigators reported that vessel dilator peptide infused subcutaneously for 14 days completely stopped the growth of human pancreatic adenocarcinomas in athymic mice. When these peptide hormones (each at 1.4 mg/min/kg bodyweight) were infused for 4 weeks, in addition to completely stopping the growth of this aggressive adenocarcinoma, vessel dilator, LANP, and kaliuretic peptide decreased human pancreatic adenocarcinoma tumor volume after 1 week by 49%, 28%, and 11%, respectively, with a 109% and 2000% increase in the tumor volume in ANP- and placebo-treated mice, respectively [53].

Immunocytochemical evaluation after removal of the human pancreatic adenocarcinomas revealed that vessel dilator, LANP, kaliuretic peptide, and ANP each localized to the nucleus and cytoplasm of the cancer cells and to the endothelium of the capillaries growing into these tumors [54]. It is of interest that all four of these peptide hormones, which inhibit DNA synthesis, localized to the nucleus. More interestingly, Vesely and colleagues have also shown that a slightly modified kaliuretic peptide given by nanotechnology can substantially decrease the activation of extracellular receptor kinase (ERK-1), a growth-promoting peptide, which is able move from the plasma membrane to the nucleus to cause proliferation. These peptide hormones may inhibit the growth of cancer cells not only by directly inhibiting DNA synthesis in the nucleus of the cancer cell but by also decreasing the activation of growth-promoting substances such as ERK-1. Vesley and coworkers also reported that vessel dilator, LANP, kaliuretic peptide, and ANP caused a similar decrease in the number of breast adenocarcinoma, squamous cell lung carcinoma, and small cell lung cancer cells [55].

Summary

The natriuretic peptides are a family of structurally related hormones with diverse biologic actions. The therapeutic potential of the natriuretic peptides extends beyond acute decompensated heart failure, and more studies are needed to define fully the true therapeutic potential of this unique family of endogenous peptides.

References

[1] Chen HH, Burnett JC Jr. The natriuretic peptides in heart failure: diagnostic and therapeutic potentials. Proc Assoc Am Physicians 1999;111:406.

[2] Forssmann W, Meyer M, Forssmann K. The renal urodilatin system: clinical implications. Cardiovas Res 2001;51:450.

[3] Sudoh T, Kangawa K, Minamino N, et al. A new natriuretic peptide in porcine brain. Nature 1988; 332:78.

[4] Vesely DL, San Miguel GI, Hassan I, et al. Atrial natriuretic hormone, vessel dilator, long-acting natriuretic hormone, and kaliuretic hormone decrease the circulating concentrations of total and free T4 and free T3 with reciprocal increase in TSH. J Clin Endocrinol Metab 2001;86:5438.

[5] Wang W, Ou Y, Shi Y. AlbuBNP, a recombinant B-type natriuretic peptide and human serum albumin fusion hormone, as a long-term therapy of congestive heart failure. Pharm Res 2004;21:2105.

[6] Cataliotti A, Schirger JA, Martin FL, et al. Oral human brain natriuretic peptide activates cyclic guanosine 3′,5′-monophosphate and decreases mean arterial pressure. Circulation 2005;112:836.

[7] Schweitz H, Vigne P, Moinier D, et al. A new member of the natriuretic peptide family is present in the venom of the green mamba (Dendroaspis angusticeps). J Biol Chem 1992;267:13928.

[8] Michel GH, Murayama N, Sada T, et al. Two N-terminally truncated forms of C-type natriuretic peptide from habu snake venom. Peptides 2000;21:609.

[9] Amininasab M, Elmi MM, Endlich N, et al. Functional and structural characterization of a novel member of the natriuretic family of peptides from the venom of Pseudocerastes persicus. FEBS Lett 2004;557:104.

[10] Fry BG, Wickramaratana JC, Lemme S, et al. Novel natriuretic peptides from the venom of the inland taipan (Oxyuranus microlepidotus): isolation, chemical and biological characterisation. Biochem Biophys Res Commun 2005;327:1011.

[11] Hidaka T, Furuya M, Tani Y, et al. Hemodynamic and neurohumoral effects of carperitide (alpha-human atrial natriuretic peptide) in dogs with low-output heart failure. Nippon Yakurigaku Zasshi 1995;105:243.

[12] Publication Committee for the Intravenous Nesiritide vs Nitroglycerin for Treatment of Decompensated Congestive Heart Failure. A randomized controlled trial. JAMA 2002;287:1531.

[13] Chen HH, Burnett JC. C-type natriuretic peptide: the endothelial component of the natriuretic peptide system. J Cardiovasc Pharmacol 1998;32(Suppl 3):S22.

[14] Chen HH, Schirger JA, Chau WL, et al. Renal response to acute neutral endopeptidase inhibition in mild and severe experimental heart failure. Circulation 1999;100:2443.

[15] Chen HH, Grantham JA, Schirger JA, et al. Subcutaneous administration of brain natriuretic peptide in experimental heart failure. J Am Coll Cardiol 2000;36:1706.

[16] Belluardo P, Cataliotti A, Bonaiuto L, et al. Lack of activation of the molecular forms of the BNP system in human grade 1 hypertension and relationship to cardiac hypertrophy. Am J Physiol Heart Circ Physiol 2006;291:H1529–35.

[17] Hawkridge AM, Heublein DM, Bergen HR 3rd, et al. Quantitative mass spectral evidence for the absence of circulating brain natriuretic peptide (BNP-32) in severe human heart failure. Proc Natl Acad Sci USA 2005;102:17442.

[18] Chen HH, Redfield MM, Nordstrom LJ, et al. Subcutaneous administration of the cardiac hormone BNP in symptomatic human heart failure. J Card Fail 2004;10:115–9.

[19] Cataliotti A, Boerrigter G, Costello-Boerrigter LC, et al. Brain natriuretic peptide enhances renal actions of furosemide and suppresses furosemide-induced aldosterone activation in experimental heart failure. Circulation 2004;109:1680.

[20] Yousef ZR, Redwood SR, Marber MS. Postinfarction left ventricular remodeling: a pathophysiological and therapeutic review. Cardiovasc Drugs Ther 2000;14:243.

[21] Cohn JN, Ferrari R, Sharpe N. Cardiac remodeling—concepts and clinical implications: a consensus paper from an international forum on cardiac remodeling. Behalf of an International Forum on Cardiac Remodeling. J Am Coll Cardiol 2000;35:569.

[22] Brunner-La Rocca HP, Kaye DM, Woods RL, et al. Effects of intravenous brain natriuretic peptide on regional sympathetic activity in patients with chronic heart failure as compared to healthy control subjects. J Am Coll Cardiol 2001;37:1221.

[23] Inoue M, Kanda T, Arai M, et al. Impaired expression of brain natriuretic peptide gene in diabetic rats with myocardial infarction. Exp Clin Endocrinol Diabetes 1998;106:484.

[24] Maeda K, Tsutamoto T, Wada A, et al. Insufficient secretion of atrial natriuretic peptide at acute phase of myocardial infarction. J Appl Physiol 2000;89:458.

[25] Hayashi M, Tsutamoto T, Wada A, et al. Intravenous atrial natriuretic peptide prevents left ventricular remodeling in patients with first anterior acute myocardial infarction. J Am Coll Cardiol 2001;37:1820.

[26] Asakura M, Jiyoong K, Minamino T, et al. Rationale and design of a large-scale trial using atrial natriuretic peptide (ANP) as an adjunct to percutaneous coronary intervention for ST-segment elevation acute myocardial infarction: Japan-Working groups of acute myocardial infarction for the reduction of Necrotic Damage by ANP (J-WIND-ANP). Circ J 2004;68:95.

[27] Antman EM, Anbe DT, Armstrong PW, et al. ACC/AHA guidelines for the management of patients with ST-elevation myocardial infarction: a report of the American College of Cardiology/American Heart Association Task Force on Practice Guidelines (Committee to Revise the 1999 Guidelines for the Management of patients with acute myocardial infarction). J Am Coll Cardiol 2004;44:E1.

[28] Chen HH, Cataliotti A, Schirger JA, et al. Equimolar doses of atrial and brain natriuretic peptides and urodilatin have differential renal actions in overt experimental heart failure. Am J Physiol Regul Integr Comp Physiol 2005;288:R1093.

[29] Margulies KB, Burnett JC Jr. Neutral endopeptidase 24.11: a modulator of natriuretic peptides. Semin Nephrol 1993;13:71.

[30] Chen H, Schirger J, Wright R, et al. Intravenous BNP at the time of acute anterior myocardial infarction in humans improves left ventricular remodeling. Circulation 2005;112(Suppl 17):II.

[31] Hayashida N, Chihara S, Tayama E, et al. Coronary artery bypass grafting in patients with mild renal insufficiency. Jpn Circ J 2001;65:28.

[32] Anderson RJ, O'Brien M, MaWhinney S, et al. Mild renal failure is associated with adverse outcome after cardiac valve surgery. Am J Kidney Dis 2000;35:1127.

[33] Valsson F, Ricksten SE, Hedner T, et al. Effects of atrial natriuretic peptide on acute renal impairment in patients with heart failure after cardiac surgery. Intensive Care Med 1996;22:230.

[34] Wang DJ, Dowling TC, Meadows D, et al. Nesiritide does not improve renal function in patients with chronic heart failure and worsening serum creatinine. Circulation 2004;110:1620.

[35] Sackner-Bernstein JD, Skopicki HA, Aaronson KD. Risk of worsening renal function with nesiritide in patients with acutely decompensated heart failure. Circulation 2005;111:1487.

[36] Marcus LE, Hart D, Packer M, et al. Hemodynamic and renal excretory effects of human brain

natriuretic peptide infusion in patients with congestive heart failure. Circulation 1996;94:3184.
[37] Mills RM, LeJemtel TH, Horton DP, et al. Sustained hemodynamic effects of an infusion of nesiritide (human b-type natriuretic peptide) in heart failure: a randomized, double-blind, placebo-controlled clinical trial. J Am Coll Cardiol 1999;34:155.
[38] Yoshimura M, Yasue H, Morita E, et al. Hemodynamic, renal, and hormonal responses to brain natriuretic peptide infusion in patients with congestive heart failure. Circulation 1991;84(4):1581–8.
[39] Riter HG, Redfield MM, Burnett JC, et al. Nonhypotensive low-dose nesiritide has differential renal effects compared with standard-dose nesiritide in patients with acute decompensated heart failure and renal dysfunction. J Am Coll Cardiol 2006; 47:2334.
[40] Sezai A, Shiono M, Orime Y, et al. Low-dose continuous infusion of human atrial natriuretic peptide during and after cardiac surgery. Ann Thorac Surg 2000;69:732.
[41] Hebeler F, Oz M. Effect of perioperative nesiritide administration on postoperative renal function and clinical outcomes in patients undergoing cardiothoracic surgery. Circulation 2006;113:e807.
[42] Sakamoto M, Nakao K, Morii N, et al. The lung as a possible target organ for atrial natriuretic polypeptide secreted from the heart. Biochem Biophys Res Commun 1986;135:515.
[43] Panchenko MV, Vinogradov AD. Interaction between the mitochondrial ATP synthetase and ATPase inhibitor protein: active/inactive slow pH-dependent transitions of the inhibitor protein. FEBS Lett 1985;184:226.
[44] Perreault T, Gutkowska J. Role of atrial natriuretic factor in lung physiology and pathology. Am J Respir Crit Care Med 1995;151:226.

[45] Gutkowska J, Nemer M. Structure, expression, and function of atrial natriuretic factor in extra-atrial tissues. Endocr Rev 1989;10:519.
[46] Vollmar AM, Schulz R. Atrial natriuretic peptide in lymphoid organs of various species. Comp Biochem Physiol A 1990;96:459.
[47] Ohbayashi H, Suito H, Takagi K. Compared effects of natriuretic peptides on ovalbumin-induced asthmatic model. Eur J Pharmacol 1998;346:55.
[48] Angus RM, McCallum MJ, Hulks G, et al. Bronchodilator, cardiovascular, and cyclic guanylyl monophosphate response to high-dose infused atrial natriuretic peptide in asthma. Am Rev Respir Dis 1993;147:1122.
[49] Fluge T, Fabel H, Wagner TO, et al. Bronchodilating effects of natriuretic and vasorelaxant peptides compared to salbutamol in asthmatics. Regul Pept 1995;59:357.
[50] Akerman MJ, Yaegashi M, Khiangte Z, et al. Bronchodilator effect of infused B-type natriuretic peptide in asthma. Chest 2006;130:66.
[51] Fluge T, Forssmann WG, Kunkel G, et al. Bronchodilation using combined urodilatin-albuterol administration in asthma: a randomized, double-blind, placebo-controlled trial. Eur J Med Res 1999;4:411.
[52] Vesely BA, McAfee Q, Gower WR Jr, et al. Four peptides decrease the number of human pancreatic adenocarcinoma cells. Eur J Clin Invest 2003;33:998.
[53] Vesely DL, Clark LC, Garces AH, et al. Novel therapeutic approach for cancer using four cardiovascular hormones. Eur J Clin Invest 2004;34:674.
[54] Saba SR, Vesely DL. Cardiac natriuretic peptides: hormones with anticancer effects that localize to nucleus, cytoplasm, endothelium, and fibroblasts of human cancers. Histol Histopathol 2006;21:775.
[55] Vesely BA, Song S, Sanchez-Ramos J, et al. Five cardiac hormones decrease the number of human small-cell lung cancer cells. Eur J Clin Invest 2005;35:388.

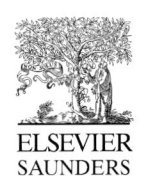

Index

Note: Page numbers of article titles are in **boldface** type.

A

Acute Decompensated Heart Failure Registry (ADHERE), 353

Acute respiratory distress syndrome, as influence on interpretation of B-type natriuretic peptide levels, 303

Acute Shortness of Breath Evaluation, B-type natriuretic peptide for (BASEL), 300–301

Age, as influence on interpretation of B-type natriuretic peptide levels, 302

Angina pectoris, stable, NT-proBNP and BNP in, 311–312

Aortic regurgitation, 349

Aortic stenosis, 348–349

Aortic valve disease, natriuretic peptides and, 348–349

Asthma therapy, natriuretic peptides in, 370

Atrial natriuretic peptide, 255, 269, 272–273, 365

B

Biomarkers, in cardiovascular diseases, 333

Blood, human, natriuretic peptides in, release and stability of, 291–292

Brain natriuretic peptide(s), 255, 269, 271, 272, 277, 365. See also Natriuretic peptide(s), B-type.
 -A, survey, 2006 College of American Pathologists, participants in, 293
 AlbuBNP, 366–367
 amino acid structure of, versus ANP, CNP, and urodilation, 296
 and N-terminal proBNP, in heart failure, 277
 and NT-proBNP, diagnostic algorithms for, 306, 307
  molecular structure and amino acid sequence of, 293, 294
  relationship of, 291, 292
 and NT-proBNP assays, correlation between manufacturers of, 294, 295
  current commercial, and cut-offs for heart failure, 293
  plasma, targets of, **291–298**
 assays, two methods compared, 294–295
 commercial assays, 293, 294
 cross-reactivities of, to other natriuretic-like peptides, 296
 or NT-proBNP, diagnostic applications of natriuretic peptides in, 318
 oral, structure of, 367
  to preserve myocardial structure and function, 273–274
 single-antibody competitive immunoassays for, 293

Breathing Not Properly trial, 300

C

Cancer therapy, natriuretic peptides in, 371

Cardiac fibroblasts, natriuretic peptides and, 271–272

Cardiac hypertrophy, in heart failure, 346

Cardiocytes, atrial, polypeptide hormones and, 255

Cardiomyocytes, function of, natriuretic peptides and, 269–271

Cardiomyopathy, patients with family history of, natriuretic peptides in screening for cardiac dysfunction in, 328–329

Cardiopulmonary bypass surgery, renal protection during, 368–370

Cardiovascular disease(s), biomarkers in, 333
 mortality in, natriuretic peptides and prediction of, 283–284
 natriuretic peptides and, 259–263
 natriuretic peptides as markers of, 284–285

Carperitide, 365

Chemotherapy, patients undergoing, natriuretic peptides in screening for cardiac dysfunction in, 328

College of American Pathologists, 2006 BNP-A survey of, participants in, 293

Congestive heart failure, left ventricle and, low levels of natriuretic peptides due to, 306–307

Coronary syndrome, acute, as influence on interpretation of B-type natriuretic peptide levels, 304–305

Coronary syndromes, acute, natriuretic peptides and, 260–261
    non-ST-elevation, early risk stratification of, 314–315
    NT-proBNP and BNP in, 312–314
    selection of treatment in, 315–317

D

Dendroaspis natriuretic peptide(s), in severe heart failure, 274

Diabetes mellitus, natriuretic peptides in screening for cardiac dysfunction in, 327–328

Dialysis, clearance of natriuretic peptides related to, 281
    estimation of hydration status in patients on, 285–286

E

Evaluation Study of Congestive Heart Failure and Pulmonary Artery Catheterization Effectiveness (ESCAPE), 353, 355

G

Gender, as influence on interpretation of B-type natriuretic peptide levels, 302

Glomerular filtration rate, stages of chronic kidney disease and, 277, 278

H

Heart, dysfunction of, screening for, natriuretic peptides in, **323–332**

Heart disease(s), ischemic, forms of, 311
    NT-proBNP and BNP in, 311–318
    valvular, natriuretic peptides in, **345–352**
        as markers of disease severity, 345–346

Heart failure, acute, diagnosis of, in renal insufficiency, 281–283
    acute decompensated, B-type natriuretic peptides in, **353–364**
        current therapies in, 354–362
        inotropic therapy in, 355
        nesiritide in, 356–359
            random trials of, 356–357
        recommendations for therapy for, 361–362
        ultrafiltration in, 355
        vasodilator therapy in, 355
    cardiac hypertrophy in, 346
    chronic, with hypertension, chronic therapy in, 366
    clinical monitoring of B-type natriuretic peptides in, **333–343**
    congestive, left ventricle and, low levels of natriuretic peptides due to, 306–307
    diagnosis of, difficulty of, 299
    natriuretic peptides, BNP and N-terminal proBNP in, 277
    previous, as influence on interpretation of B-type natriuretic peptide levels, 301–302
    severe, dendroaspis natriuretic peptide in, 274

Heart Failure Society of America, acute decompensated heart failure and, 354

High-output status, as influence on interpretation of B-type natriuretic peptide levels, 304–305

Human recombinant atrial natriuretic peptide, 365

Hypertension, chronic heart failure with, chronic therapy in, 366
    patients with, natriuretic peptides in screening for cardiac dysfunction in, 328

K

Kidneys, chronic disease of, levels of natriuretic peptides in, 278–279
        with no evidence of heart failure, 278, 279
        stages of, glomerular filtration rate and, 277, 278
    failure of, as influence on interpretation of B-type natriuretic peptide levels, 303–304
    insufficiency of. See *Renal insuciency.*
    protection of, during cardiopulmonary bypass surgery, 368–370
    role in clearance of natriuretic peptides, 279–281

Knockout mice natriuretic peptide receptor A, 270

L

Lung disease, with right heart failure, as influence on interpretation of B-type natriuretic peptide levels, 303

M

Matrix metalloproteinases, 273–274

Mitral regurgitation, 347–348

Mitral stenosis, rheumatic, 346–347

Mitral valve diseases, natriuretic peptides and, 346–347

Myocardial cell origin C-type natriuretic peptide, 365

Myocardial infarction, acute, natriuretic peptide therapy in, 273
    adverse left ventricular remodeling following, prevention of, 367–368
    natriuretic peptides in screening for cardiac dysfunction in, 327
    ST-elevation, 317–318

Myocardium, structure and function of, natriuretic peptides as regulators of, **269–276**

N

Natriuretic peptide(s), and aortic valve disease, 348–349
    and cardiac fibroblasts, 271–272
    and cardiomyocyte function, 269–271
    and cardiovascular disease, 259–263
    and mitral valve diseases, 346–347
    and prediction of mortality in cardiovascular disease, 283–284
    and renal insufficiency, clinical significance of, and role of renal clearance, **277–290**
    appropriate cut-off values for, 318–319
    as diagnostic test, **299–309**
    as markers of cardiovascular disease, 284–285
    as regulators of myocardial structure and function, **269–276**
    as screening markers for heart failure, challenges in, 323–325
        prequisites for, 324
    atrial, 255, 269, 272–273, 365
        human recombinant, 365
    B-type, and N-terminal fragment of pro B-type natriuretic peptide, 299
        in acute decompensated heart failure, **353–364**
        in heart failure, clinical monitoring of, **333–343**
        prediction of response to therapy of, 338
        interpretation of levels of, comorbidities influencing, 301–305
    peptide/NT-proB-type natriuretic peptide(s) and, levels of, 334
        and hemodynamic indices, 334–335
        and monitoring in other settings, 339
        changes in response to treatment, 337–338
        intraindividual variation in, 335–337
        serial monitoring of, 337
        therapy guided by, 338–339
    synthesis and secretion of, 333–334
    brain. See *Brain natriuretic peptide(s); Natriuretic peptide(s), B-type.*
    clearance of, kidneys in, 279–281
    commercial diagnostic assays for, characteristics of, 294
        history of, 292
    deficiencies of, in cardiovascular disease, 272–273
    dendroaspis, in severe heart failure, 274
    diagnostic applications of, in ischemic heart disease, **311–321**
        NT-proBNP or BNP in, 318
        timing of measurement of, 320
    dialysis-related clearance of, 281
    existing and novel forms of therapeutic potential for, **365–373**
    for diagnosis of acute congestive heart failure, studies of, 300–301
    forms of, in human blood, release and stability of, 291–292
    gene expression of, 255, 257
        hemodynamic and neurohumoral determinants of, 259
        processing, and slection of, diagnostic implications of, **255–268**
    in acute coronary syndromes, 260–261
    in asthma therapy, 370
    in cancer therapy, 371
    in humans, family of, 365
    in screening for cardiac dysfunction, **323–332**
        assay variability and, 325
        at-risk patient populations for, 327–329
        biologic variability of, 324–325
        optimal screening strategies for, 325–326
        population screening for, 326–327
        target definition variability and, 325
    in valvular heart diseases, **345–352**
        as markers of disease severity, 345–346
    interaction with profibrotic cytokine transforming growth factor-beta, 271

Natriuretic peptide(s) (*continued*)
　levels in chronic kidney disease, 278–279
　　with no evidence of heart failure, 278, 279
　low levels of, conditions causing, 305–307
　metabolism and clearance of, 279–280
　pathophysiologic and physiologic importance of, 255
　physiologic properties of, and therapeutic potential of, 365–366
　processing of, 256, 258
　production of, 279
　secretion of, basal, 256
　　stimulated, 256–257
　structure of, 365
　testing of, in renal insufficiency, clinical significance of, 281–286
　to preserve myocardial structure and function, therapeutic implications for, 273–274

Natriuretic peptide receptor A, 255, 269
　biology of, 270
　dominant negative form of, 270
　knockout mice, 270

Nesiritide, actions of, 356
　as therapeutic application of B-type natriuretic peptides, 355–356
　in acute decompensated heart failure, 356–359
　　random trials of, 356–357
　recommendations for use of, 362
　risk-benefit profile of, 359–361

NT-proBNP, and brain natriuretic peptides, diagnostic algorithms for, 306, 307
　molecular structure and amino sequence of, 293, 294
　relationship of, 291, 292
　or brain natriuretic peptide, diagnostic applications of natriuretic peptides in, 318

NT-proBNP assays, and brain natriuretic assays, correlation between manufacturers of, 294, 295
　current commercial, and cut-offs for heart failure, 293
　plasma, targets of, **291–298**

O

Obesity, low levels of natriuretic peptides due to, 305

P

Peptide(s), natriuretic. See *Natriuretic peptide(s)*.

Polypeptide hormones, cardiocytes in atria and, 255

ProBNP Investigation of Dyspnea in Emergency Department (PRIDE), 301

Profibrotic cytokine transforming growth factor-beta, natriuretic peptide interaction with, 271

Prospective Randomized Evaluation of Cardiac Ectopy with Dobutamine or Natrecor Therapy (PRESCEDENT) study, 358

Prospective Randomized Outcomes of Acute Congestive Heart Failure Treated Initially as Outpatients with Nesiritide (PROACTION), 358–359

Pulmonary disease, as influence on interpretation of B-type natriuretic peptide levels, 302–303

Pulmonary edema, flash, low levels of natriuretic peptides due to, 306

Pulmonary embolism, as influence on interpretation of B-type natriuretic peptide levels, 303

R

Rapid Emergency Department Heart Failure Outpatient Trial (REDHOT), 301, 302

Renal insufficiency, and natriuretic peptides, clinical significance of, and role of renal clearance, **277–290**
　diagnosis of, acute heart failure in, 281–283
　natriuretic peptide testing in, clinical significance of, 281–286
　natriuretic peptides in screening for cardiac dysfunction in, 328

Rheumatic mitral stenosis, 346–347

U

Ultrafiltration versus IV Diuretics for Patients Hospitalized for Acute Decompensated Congestive Heart Failure (UNLOAD), 355

V

Vasodilation in Management of Acute Congestive Heart Failure (VMAC) trial, 358

Moving?

Make sure your subscription moves with you!

To notify us of your new address, find your **Clinics Account Number** (located on your mailing label above your name), and contact customer service at:

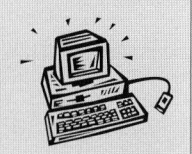

E-mail: elspcs@elsevier.com

800-654-2452 (subscribers in the U.S. & Canada)
407-345-4000 (subscribers outside of the U.S. & Canada)

Fax number: 407-363-9661

Elsevier Periodicals Customer Service
6277 Sea Harbor Drive
Orlando, FL 32887-4800

*To ensure uninterrupted delivery of your subscription, please notify us at least 4 weeks in advance of move.

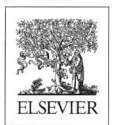

ELSEVIER